From **THE HOSPITAL FOR SICK CHILDREN**

Get a
Healthy Weight
for Your Child

A Parent's Guide to Better Eating and Exercise

Dr. Brian W. McCrindle, MD, MPH, FRCP(C)   **James G. Wengle,** MSc

Robert
ROSE

The authors would like to thank the following for sharing their knowledge and expertise during the writing of this book: Debra Katzman (MD, FRCP), Jennifer Gibson (BASc, RD), Gareth Smith (MSc), Patrick Glasgow (BSc), Andria Boulfon, Christine McDonald (BSc), Geraldine Cullen-Dean (RN, MN) — and CIBC World Markets Children's Miracle Foundation for financial support.

This book is a general guide only and should never be a substitute for the skill, knowledge, and experience of a qualified medical professional dealing with the facts, circumstances, and symptoms of a particular case.

The nutritional, medical, and health information presented in this book is based on the research, training, and professional experience of the authors, and is true and complete to the best of their knowledge. However, this book is intended only as an informative guide for those wishing to know more about health, nutrition, and medicine; it is not intended to replace or countermand the advice given by the reader's personal physician. Because each person and situation is unique, the authors and the publisher urge the reader to check with a qualified health-care professional before using any procedure where there is a question as to its appropriateness. A physician should be consulted before beginning any exercise program. The authors and the publisher are not responsible for any adverse effects or consequences resulting from the use of the information in this book. It is the responsibility of the reader to consult a physician or other qualified health-care professional regarding his or her personal care.

**Library and Archives Canada
Cataloguing in Publication**

McCrindle, Brian W.
  Get a healthy weight for your child :
a parent's guide to better eating and exercise /
Brian W. McCrindle, James G. Wengle.

Includes index.
ISBN 0-7788-0114-4

1. Obesity in children—Prevention. 2. Children—
Nutrition. 3. Exercise for children. I. Wengle,
James G. (James Gordon), 1975– II. Title.

RJ399.C6M33 2005   613.2'083   C2005-902587-5

Printed and bound in Canada.

1 2 3 4 5 6 7 8 9 CPL 13 12 11 10 09 08 07 06 05

Edited by Bob Hilderley, Senior Editor, Health
Copyedited by Fina Scroppo
Design and page composition by
    PageWave Graphics Inc.
Exercise illustrations by Kveta
Index by Martha Ayim

The publisher acknowledges the financial support of the Government of Canada through the Book Publishing Industry Development Program.

Published by Robert Rose Inc.,
120 Eglinton Ave. E., Suite 800,
Toronto, Ontario, Canada M4P 1E2
Tel: (416) 322-6552 Fax: (416) 322-6936

Contents

Get a Healthy Weight for Your Child

This book will help you to:

- Recognize if your child is overweight
- Realize the medical and emotional consequences of being overweight
- Understand the social, behavioral, biological, and genetic causes of being overweight
- Improve your child's and your family's eating habits and physical fitness

This book features:

- Practical guidelines for treatment and prevention
- Hands-on worksheets and exercises
- Food charts, menu suggestions, and exercise routines
- Charts for calculating overweight and healthy weight
- Guided nutrition tours of the fresh and processed food sections of grocery stores
- Menu plans and food preparation advice
- Strength and flexibility exercise routines
- Helpful food and fitness tips for parents
- Nutrition and activity 3-day diaries and scorecards
- Guidelines for setting weekly nutrition and activity goals

The Healthy Weight Program Summary

Program Aims

The Healthy Weight Program will help your children make the necessary changes to their nutrition and lifestyle so they become healthy and fit. The program will benefit your children if they are not at a healthy weight, if they are at risk of becoming overweight, or if they just eat poorly and are physically unfit, regardless of their weight.

Program Philosophy

A healthy weight is the weight your child's body achieves with healthy nutrition and healthy activity habits. The program is not a weight-loss diet. It will be different for each child, and there is no one specific number that your child needs to reach. So long as young people adopt a healthy lifestyle, their body will find its own healthy weight.

- **Health cannot be measured on a scale:** The most important message you can send to your child is that the goal is not weight loss. The goal of this program is good nutrition and developing an active lifestyle. As young people move closer to the eating habits and physical activity outlined in the program, their body will naturally develop a healthy weight over a healthy amount of time.
- **Healthy lifestyle can be measured:** A healthy lifestyle is one where nutritious food is eaten on a regular basis and a meaningful amount of physical activity is performed each day. The program provides the means to measure and record if children are eating nutritiously and if they are getting a meaningful amount of physical activity.

Program Principles

The program is based on the principle of balancing food energy intake and physical activity energy expenditure to achieve a healthy weight.

- **Healthy Energy Rule:** When the amount of energy from the food we eat is balanced exactly with the amount of energy the body needs to stay alive and carry out activity, our body will maintain the same amount of stored body fat. This is the state of healthy weight.
- **Positive Energy Rule:** When the amount of energy from the food we eat is more than the amount of energy the body needs to stay alive and carry out activity, our body will store the extra energy as fat. This is the state of increasing body fat.
- **Negative Energy Rule:** When the amount of energy our body needs to stay alive and carry out activity is more than the amount of energy we get from the food we eat, our body simply uses up stored fat as its energy source. This is the state of decreasing body fat.

Program Stages

Your child will take small manageable steps toward healthy nutrition and healthy activity habits by choosing weekly nutrition and activity goals. By taking these steps, your child will start adopting a healthy lifestyle and will become physically fit and achieve a healthy weight.

The healthy weight program follows four stages of development. Parent and child have specific knowledge and activity goals to complete in each stage.

STAGE 1: *Assessing Nutrition and Activity Levels (Week 1)*
- Family Nutrition and Activity Habits Worksheet
- Child's Nutrition and Activity Habits Worksheet
- 3-Day Nutrition Diary: Log and Scorecard
- 3-Day Activity Diary: Log and Scorecard
- Height, Weight, and Target Weight Chart

STAGE 2: *Setting Goals and Rewards (Week 2)*
- Goal of the Week Worksheet
- Goal of the Week Evaluation Questionnaire
- 3-Day Nutrition Diary: Log and Scorecard
- 3-Day Activity Diary: Log and Scorecard

STAGE 3: *Building Up Goals and Rewards (Week 3-4)*
- Goal of the Week Worksheet
- Goal of the Week Evaluation Questionnaire
- 3-Day Nutrition Diary: Log and Scorecard
- 3-Day Activity Diary: Log and Scorecard
- Height, Weight, and Target Weight Chart

STAGE 4: *Maintaining Progress (Beyond Week 4)*
Weekly
- Goal of the Week Worksheet
- Goal of the Week Evaluation Questionnaire

Monthly
- 3-Day Nutrition Diary: Log and Scorecard
- 3-Day Activity Diary: Log and Scorecard
- Family Nutrition and Activity Habits Worksheet
- Child's Nutrition and Activity Habits Worksheet

Biweekly
- Height, Weight, and Target Weight Chart

Introduction

James' Story

June 10, 1993! That was the day. The day that ended up changing my life. I have never needed to memorize the date. It just sticks in my mind. So do the numbers: 5'11", 210 pounds, and 38 inches. As you will learn while reading this book, at a height of 5'11", 210 pounds is considerably overweight even for a 17-year-old. And a waist size of 38 is very worrying. On June 10, I took the first step on a road to an entirely different lifestyle.

My name is James (my friends call me Jay), and I am a middle child in a family with four siblings. I grew up with two parents who always gave me unconditional love and support in whatever I attempted. As a young child, I was very active and, physically, I was lean. Excess body fat only became an issue for me in grade school when my level of physical activity started to decline and my food choices became poorer.

Food as Love

Growing up in an indulgent family, my siblings and I were always provided with anything we needed. Part of the love we were shown was expressed with food. Sunday was family day. Dinner on Sunday night was always a feast and always involved lots of desserts. During the rest of the week, we ate prepared meals, leftovers, and prepackaged and frozen dinners. Both my parents worked, so it was difficult for them to make a new meal each night. According to my older siblings, my younger sister and I got much more junk cereal, junk snack food, and fast food than they had growing up. This was probably because my parents worked longer hours when the family grew and money was tight.

According to my older siblings, my younger sister and I got much more junk cereal, junk snack food, and fast food than they had growing up.

My Sweet Tooth

My big sweet tooth was also responsible for much of the junk food we had because my parents had trouble saying no to my requests. I always convinced my dad that I needed to buy fast food after my soccer games and that I needed extra money beyond my weekly allowance to buy candy. Throughout my entire childhood, I had no knowledge about nutrition and health. I probably didn't care either. How many kids do? I can't even remember being taught the basics of Canada's Food Guide in school. Our house was often stocked with junk cereal and other junk food. My appetite and my sweet tooth made sure that junk food didn't last more than a week in our house. In fact, even when my mom bought extra it was still gone in the same amount of time.

Junk Food

The corner store was one of my favorite places, and I went there often to buy chips and chocolate bars. I loved McDonald's chicken McNuggets, too. McDonald's was my favorite 'restaurant' to visit. I always ordered nine chicken nuggets because six was never enough. I also dipped them in loads of sweet-and-sour sauce and used the sauce for dipping my fries as well. Then I washed it all down with my orange drink. That's not all. I also loved baking, and when I did, I ate much of what I baked. My food environment contributed to the weight gain I experienced as I got older. But there was an additional reason for my unhealthy weight gain — that was my level of activity.

Changing Shape

In my early school years I was fairly active. Even in the winter, I spent a lot of time outside and I skied every weekend. In the spring, I played soccer and, in the summer, I went to camp. I also walked to school every day. At school, I was active in gym class, and my two recess periods and lunch break were spent running around the school grounds. I grew quickly throughout early grade school and was the tallest in my class, but by Grade 6, I wasn't growing as fast. That was when my food environment began to affect me. The weight started accumulating and, to make matters worse, I started spending more time on the computer and in front of the television and less time outside.

I grew quickly throughout early grade school and was the tallest in my class, but by Grade 6, I wasn't growing as fast. That was when my food environment began to affect me.

Slowing Down

As I gained weight, I had more trouble doing physical activity. I would feel out of breath, and that discouraged me from participating. I also started becoming more aware of my body size, and I wanted to do something about it. My dad was always into sports and he ran regularly, so I decided to try running with him. Having him as a role model was very helpful, but my attempts at running didn't last long. I was having trouble breathing after running for a few minutes, and that was uncomfortable and scary for me. I was probably starting off too quickly and trying to run too far. The difficulty I had with breathing discouraged me, so I gave up trying. I also had difficulties in gym class at school, where I found myself being short of breath when running around.

By the time I got to high school, my weight was more apparent. This created more embarrassing problems. I had an interest in participating in school athletics and I really wanted to improve my fitness, but I ran into lots of obstacles. I always avoided team sports because I was too worried that we might play shirts against skins and that people would see my body. I was also deathly afraid of changing in front of my peers. These fears made it difficult for me to participate in most sports. For the same reasons, swimming was also a challenge. I would claim that wearing a shirt kept me warm when I went swimming at friends' houses.

I always avoided team sports because I was too worried that we might play shirts against skins and that people would see my body. I was also deathly afraid of changing in front of my peers.

The Cycle Continues...

My poor food environment, combined with less physical activity, led to an initial gain in weight that affected my ability to perform physical activity and encouraged inactivity. This led to more weight gain, poorer physical fitness, and fears of how people looked at my body. The cycle continued.

Teasing at Home

Being overweight wasn't only affecting me physically. I also had to deal with a fair share of teasing. It was never my parents; they were always supportive. I can't remember ever feeling that they judged me by my weight. It was never even an issue with them. I guess they didn't notice the changes in my weight because they saw me all the time. I never really talked to them about how I felt about my appearance. Now, when they look back at pictures, they're able to see that I was struggling with my weight.

My siblings, on the other hand, were more aware. I remember once teasing my younger sister and receiving a comeback that hit hard. She looked at me and said, "At least I'm not fat!" That was the first time my younger sister had found words that could make me cry. Another experience hurt even more. My brother is 10 years older than I am. He was my hero as a child. When we were growing up, I never stopped annoying him, and he never let me get away with this. I respected him very much. One day, as I was innocently leaning back in a chair, he looked at me, saw my stomach, and said, "You're fat!" That hurt much more than a comment coming from my younger sister could. I fought hard to keep the tears back as a lump filled my throat. Nothing hurts more than an insult from someone you respect and look up to.

Teasing Away from Home

Teasing from outside the home also had an impact. I still remember how it felt when I was mistaken for a girl while looking for a gift card with my mom. The salesperson asked my mom if the card was for her daughter's friend. School also provided its share of embarrassing moments. I distinctly remember being prodded in the belly and being called a "Pillsbury Doughboy." My experiences with being overweight were not good ones. The desire to do something about it grew and grew.

The Turning Point

The best decision I ever made in high school was to take a senior level phys-ed class with Mr. Bos. He taught a class where the focus was on education about physical activity, health, and nutrition. There was a physical component as well, but it never required me to remove my shirt. The class was only 5 months long but it changed my life forever.

From our phys-ed teacher, we learned a lot about the science of physical activity and nutrition and how they lead to good health. We were taught all about the health benefits of strength training, endurance activities, and good nutrition. For the final month of the class, each student was responsible for bringing a guest speaker to talk about a health-related topic. It was because of a guest speaker discussing nutrition that I came home from school on June 10, 1993 and proclaimed to my parents, "Today is the Day."

Becoming Self-Aware

My phys-ed class taught me important basic concepts about nutrition and physical activity. Taking the class also made me self-aware. I knew that I was overweight because of how I felt doing physical activity and because of measurements we had taken. At one point, we were asked to keep track of our eating for a few days. I discovered that I was eating too many foods that were high in energy and low in nutrition. We also kept records of our physical activity. This allowed us to keep track of the amount of time we spent doing endurance activity and strength training. Using the records, we could also see any improvements we were making. My physical activity level was very low and my performance was poor compared with the other students. I also knew that I was not fit because of the way I felt when running even short distances. Because I knew what my own specific problem areas were in nutrition and physical activity, I understood what I needed to work on to be healthy.

Making Changes

My parents were very supportive when I came home that first day proclaiming that I was going to make a change. I wanted to work on my nutrition and physical activity at the same time. They both agreed to help me. To improve my nutrition, I needed by mom's support because she did the shopping and prepared many of the meals in the house. For physical activity, having my dad as a role model was extremely helpful. I felt that there was no reason why I couldn't be physically active and fit just like him. I decided to try my luck at running again. When I had tried taking up running with my dad and other friends before, I had encountered difficulties. Either my breathing got in the way or my knees hurt. Now I know that both of those problems were caused by excess weight.

My parents were very supportive when I came home that first day proclaiming that I was going to make a change.

Doing It Right

I approached my goal of running differently this time. The first difference was that I bought shoes that were meant for running and provided me with adequate support. The second difference was how I actually set out to achieve my goal. Instead of trying to match the level of my dad or my friends, who were regular runners, I worked at my own pace. The first run I made toward my goal was only one loop around my street. This was as far as I could go before I had difficulty breathing. It only took about 3 minutes and the distance was less than half a kilometer. That didn't matter, though — what did matter was that the next night I ran again. I kept track of how many times I went around my street and how long it took. It was easy to keep track — the first week the number was always one. I didn't try to advance too quickly. I only added another loop of the street when I felt ready. The important thing was that I kept going and kept setting my goals a tiny bit higher. In addition, I had a longer-term goal. I desperately wanted to run a 10-km race. This was a lofty goal when I could barely complete a few laps around my street, but I kept it in the back of my mind.

Measuring Up to Success

Instead of using a scale regularly to measure my weight, I used several other methods to make sure I was on the right track. I used the distance I was able to run and my waist size as my main measures. For me, weight was an unreliable measure in the short term because when I measured on a daily basis, it sometimes went up and sometimes went down. I decided to measure my weight and waist size every couple of weeks so that I wouldn't be bothered if the change was too small to see. I was never concerned with the actual number on the scale, only that I was moving in the right direction. One thing I noticed, though, was that even though my running performance steadily improved, my waist size and weight sometimes showed great changes and other times they stayed the same for a while before changing again. I had started another growth spurt during this time and that was probably partly responsible for the sporatic improvements.

I decided to measure my weight and waist size every couple of weeks so that I wouldn't be bothered if the change was too small to see.

Keeping at It

After making my first measurements of waist size and weight, I decided to stop making any measurements until 1 month after the start of my new lifestyle. I guessed that it would take this long for a noticeable change to occur. I don't remember what I weighed after that month, but I do know that my waist size had shrunk by one whole inch. This was incredibly motivating for me because it meant that all of my efforts were paying off. It also gave me a better idea of how long it would take for me to get to a healthier size. The success drove me to carry on with determination and confidence.

Setbacks

Unfortunately, an accident threatened to undo all my hard work. While playing football with some friends, I rolled my ankle very badly. The injury meant that I had to give up running for a while. Even walking was difficult for me. I was extremely upset and worried. Instead of giving up on all I had accomplished, I focused on what I could do rather than on what I couldn't. I became a little more careful about the number of treats I allowed myself and I started using a rowing machine, which put less pressure on my aching ankle. When the pain and swelling decreased in my ankle, I also started walking loops around my street. I slowly added light jogs every now and again. It did take some time to get back to the level I had achieved before the accident, but I did eventually get there and was once again on the path to a healthier weight.

Real Change

After a summer of healthy eating and physical activity, I had lost a considerable amount of weight. In fact, some people who hadn't seen me over the summer didn't even recognize me.

In the spring, I finally achieved one of my long-term goals. I enrolled in my first 10 km race and I successfully completed it.

I continued eating healthy and running during that fall and into the winter. Winter was a real challenge because running in below zero temperature can be difficult and uncomfortable. I dressed properly and I adapted to breathing in the cold air. The real test of my physical fitness came on a family skiing trip. We returned to the same place we had been two years before. Breathing difficulties and constant headaches had gotten in the way of skiing on the previous trip. On this trip, I had no problems at all. I even indulged in some less nutritious foods on the trip. This was not a problem, though, because when I returned from the trip, I returned to eating nutritiously. In the spring, I finally achieved one of my long-term goals. I enrolled in my first 10-km race and I successfully completed it.

Confidence

From that spring onward, I have never been teased about my weight, and I have the confidence to partake in physical activities. My experiences have helped me develop confidence in my ability to set goals and achieve them even if they are lofty and far off in the distance. The self-esteem I developed through my accomplishments also gave me confidence when socializing with others outside of physical activity.

Permanent Changes

Since changing my lifestyle more than 10 years ago, I have developed a keen interest in health, nutrition, and exercise. In university, I fed those interests by taking courses in all of these subjects. I also maintained my healthy eating habits and my level of physical activity. These habits are just a natural part of my lifestyle now, and I still get great pleasure from being able to succeed at physically demanding activities. There are times, now and then, when I am less physically active and there are times when I eat less nutritiously. Even so, I stay at a healthy weight. The biggest reason I maintain a healthy lifestyle is because of the way it makes me feel. During times when I'm less active, I actually feel like I have less energy and I also feel less capable of meeting physical challenges. When I'm active, I feel energetic, confident, and full of life.

The biggest reason I maintain a healthy lifestyle is because of the way it makes me feel. During times when I'm less active, I actually feel like I have less energy and I also feel less capable of meeting physical challenges.

Helping Others

My experience as an overweight teenager has given me personal understanding of how being overweight can make a person feel. I know about the physical and emotional struggles. Even though I had role models when I was growing up, I never had a personal mentor who saw my potential and helped guide me toward a healthy lifestyle. I had to believe in myself and find my own way. I did learn a great deal about myself and about my own abilities in the process, but I definitely could have benefited from outside encouragement and recognition of my small successes along the way. If my weight gain had been noticed before the physical problems set in, maybe my experience in high school would have been as favorable as my experience at university. Through my own experiences with being overweight and overcoming it, I'm hopeful that I can help other children do the same. I have great compassion for children and I will always aspire to help them in whatever I do.

My experience as an overweight teenager has given me personal understanding of how being overweight can make a person feel. I know about the physical and emotional struggles.

— James Wengle

The Healthy Weight Program

We have developed a program to help parents ensure that their children are healthy and fit so that they don't experience the medical and social consequences of being overweight. Many aspects of the program are very similar to the way in which James successfully managed his own weight problem.

In order to help your child use the program successfully, you will need to spend some time learning how to use it yourself. We provide you with research into the causes and consequences of being overweight, as well medical information about good nutrition and healthy physical activity, before putting this information into action in a step-by-step practical program. Once you have a good grasp of how the program works, you can introduce it to your children so that your son or daughter can follow these steps toward achieving a healthier lifestyle and a healthy body weight.

Start Early

Managing children's eating habits is most effective while they are young. From infancy to late childhood, children are developing their eating and activity habits. These nutrition and exercise habits will carry them into adulthood. On the one hand, if young children start by eating poorly and exercising very little, it may be extremely difficult to change this course as they get older. On the other hand, exposing your children to healthy eating habits and providing opportunities for physical activity when they are younger will make them much more likely to continue eating healthy and participating in physical activity right into adulthood.

Young children are less likely to question changes in the quality of food you provide them. They may go through a phase in adolescence where they become less concerned about their health, but they will fall back on their deep-rooted healthy habits as they become mature. Helping your child develop healthy habits at an earlier age will be easier for you and for them.

Be a Role Model

As a parent, you will be most influential while your children are young. You are their role model during these early years. How you eat and your level of physical activity will have an enduring impact on their lives. As your children begin to

---

Program Aim

The Healthy Weight Program will help your children make the necessary changes to their nutrition and lifestyle so they become healthy and fit. The program will benefit your children if they are not at a healthy weight, if they are at risk of becoming overweight, or if they just eat poorly and are physically unfit, regardless of their weight.

develop independence, they often become less influenced by your choices and instructions while their peers become more influential. Even then, you can become a role model by making good food choices and exercising regularly. Parents have a greater impact on adolescents by 'doing what they say' rather than saying what their child should do. The Healthy Weight Program should, ideally, be followed by parent and child and the entire family, if possible, to be most effective.

Case Histories

To help you in becoming a role model and to let you see how other parents have coped with the problem of having an overweight child in the family, we have provided several case histories that run throughout the book. These histories are composites of actual cases we have treated in our clinics at The Hospital for Sick Children. Sometimes medical professionals become too abstract and clinical in their explanation of health problems; these case histories make these problems immediate and personal. They should speak to you as you lead your child to getting a healthy weight.

Qualifications

The information presented in this book is based on the most current research in pediatric nutrition, exercise, and overweight disorders. The Healthy Weight Program derives from this research and our clinical experience at The Hospital for Sick Children. The combination of our expertise and experience offers a unique perspective on the problem of overweight and a down-to-earth approach to solving it. Dr. Brian McCrindle is a senior scientist and cardiologist in the Division of Cardiology at The Hospital for Sick Children and Professor of Pediatrics at the University of Toronto. James Wengle, who studied for his Master of Science degree at the University of Guelph, overcame childhood obesity and is now committed to parent education and prevention of this condition. Members of the pediatric team at The Hospital for Sick Children have also contributed vital information and recommendations to the content of this book.

CHAPTER 1

How Serious Is the Overweight Problem?

The problem of children being overweight, even obese, has become headline news, discussed in homes, at schools, and among medical professionals. We have been cautioned that overweight children may be at risk of developing life-threatening health conditions, such as high blood pressure, heart disease, and type 2 diabetes, conditions we typically associate with middle and older age, not with youth. Despite some naysayers who suggest that studies linking overweight in children with serious health problems is 'crying wolf', there is good reason for attending to the problem of overweight in children and for helping your children achieve a healthy weight. A quick review of the best medical research into this problem shows why following a healthy weight program makes sense. This review should answer your most frequently asked questions about overweight and obesity in children. Rest assured that despite the disturbing statistics and studies, your child can achieve a healthy weight and long-term good health.

Five Facts About Children's Overweight

1. Overweight in children has been proven to have important long-term health consequences.

2. Overweight in children can affect their self-esteem, self-image, self-confidence, and emotional well-being.

3. Improper eating habits, poor nutrition, and lack of physical activity, combined with increases in sedentary recreation, contribute to overweight in children.

4. Overweight is caused by an energy imbalance, where more calories are consumed than are used by the body, with the excess calories being stored as fat.

5. Genetics or heredity may have an effect on an individual's energy balance, causing a person to be more or less likely to become overweight.

CASE STUDY Anne's Family

A Visit to the Doctor

"High cholesterol!" Anne exclaimed. "How could he have high cholesterol?" Her 11-year-old son, Cody, shifted anxiously. Anne had brought Cody to the doctor 2 weeks ago because he had been having stomach pains, and the doctor had done some routine blood tests. The doctor also explained that Cody's liver tests were abnormal, and that both of these problems were probably related to Cody's weight. The doctor mentioned a condition called fatty liver that some children with obesity can have, which could also lead to liver damage in some cases. He was going to schedule Cody to have an ultrasound test of his liver.

The doctor told Anne and Cody that these were only some of the health problems that very overweight children can have. If Cody did not start to lose some weight and lead a healthy lifestyle, the problems would only get worse.

continued on page 29

A Growing Problem

The statistics are staggering that show the increase in overweight and obesity among adults and children during the past 25 years, primarily in North America, but also in other Western countries or countries being "westernized."

Q: **What's the difference between being 'overweight' and 'obese'?**

A: Many terms have been used while trying to describe excess body fat in adults and in children. The terms can have different meanings in different countries and among different health researchers and medical doctors. While summarizing research findings, we will keep the original terms used by the researchers. Throughout the remainder of the book we will use the term overweight to describe children with excess body fat. We find 'overweight' to be less hurtful than 'obese' and less technical than 'at risk', a term used by some medical professionals.seems to be more strongly related to increased waist size than to other measures of obesity.

North America

In Canada alone, from 1985 to 1998, the percentage of adults who were obese (more extreme than just overweight) rose from 5.6% to 14.8%, which meant that in 1998, 3.3 million Canadians were obese. At that rate, half of all adults would be obese by 2033. The Canadian Community Health Survey of 2001 showed that 32% of adults are overweight, while 15% are obese.

The trend affects children as well. In a survey performed in 1994-1995 and again in 1998-1999, the percentage of children aged 2 to 11 years who were classified as overweight rose from 34% to 37%, while those who were obese increased from 16% to 18%. The survey also showed that boys were more overweight than girls, with only 38% of obese children being active compared to 47% of those who were not obese.

The trends are similar in the United States. Obesity in adults rose from 12% in 1991 to 19.8% in 2000. From national surveys performed in 1988-1994 and again in 1999-2000, the percentage of overweight rose from 10.5% to 15.5% in children aged 12 to 19, from 11.3% to 15.3% in children aged 6 to 11, and from 7.2% to 10.4% in children aged 2 to 5 years.

 FACT

Pre-School Plight

Imagine, 1 in 10 pre-school children being overweight! Statistics suggest that the percentage of children with obesity has increased by four-fold in the last 25 years, affecting both boys and girls, all ages and all races.

Changes in the Prevalence of Overweight and Obesity among Canadian Adults and Children between 1981 and 1996

| | ADULTS (20-64) | | | | CHILDREN (7-13) | | | |
| | In 1981 | | In 1996 | | In 1981 | | In 1996 | |
	Males	Females	Males	Females	Boys	Girls	Boys	Girls
Overweight	48%	30%	57%	35%	15%	15%	29%	24%
Obesity	9%	8%	14%	12%	5%	5%	14%	12%

Sources: 1981 Canada Fitness Survey, 1996 National Longitudinal Survey of Children and Youth and 1996 National Population Health Survey.

Worldwide Obesity

Although definitions of overweight and obesity vary from study to study and country to country, the trends are evident worldwide. According to the World Health Organization, more than one billion adults in the world are overweight, and of these, 300 million are considered obese. The numbers are growing.

Changes in the Prevalence of Overweight Children of Various Ages in Select Countries Around the World

Canada 1981-1996 7 to 13 year-olds **15% ⟶ 27%**	United States 1994-2000 6 to 11 year-olds **11.3% ⟶ 15.3**	Australia 1985-1995 7 to 15 year-olds **1.3% ⟶ 5.1%**	Morocco 1987-1992 0 to 5 year-olds **2.7% ⟶ 6.8%**
Egypt 1978-1996 0 to 5 year-olds **2.2% ⟶ 8.6%**	Haiti 1978-1995 0 to 5 year-olds **0.8% ⟶ 2.8%**	Brazil 1974-1997 6 to 9 year-olds **4.9% ⟶ 17.4%**	Costa Rica 1982-1996 0 to 6 year-olds **2.3% ⟶ 6.2%**
England From 1984-1994 4 to 11 year-olds **1.0% ⟶ 2.1%**	Scotland From 1984-1994 4 to 11 year-olds **1.4% ⟶ 2.7%**	Japan From 1970-1996 10 year-olds **4.0% ⟶ 10.0%**	China From 1991-1997 6 to 9 year-olds **10.5% ⟶ 11.3%**

Q: **Are clothes getting smaller or are children getting bigger?**

A: A British study found waist measurements in school children were significantly larger in 1996-1998 compared to in the late 1970s and 1980s. The waistlines have continued to swell, such that by 2001, children's waists were on average 4 centimeters or two clothing sizes larger than they had been 20 years ago. Waist measurements have increased faster than other measures of overweight, suggesting that children are getting fatter around the middle than elsewhere, particularly in girls. The association between obesity and chronic disease seems to be more strongly related to increased waist size than to other measures of obesity.

Medical Consequences

Overweight during childhood and particularly during adolescence is related to increased diseases and risk of death in later life. The Harvard Growth Study looked at 508 adolescents from 1922 to 1935, and continued to follow them throughout their lives. Those boys (but not girls) who were overweight as adolescents had almost double the risk of death as adults 55 years later, with a more than two times greater risk of death from heart attack. Both overweight boys and girls had an increased risk of heart disease, with an additional increased risk of intestinal cancer and gout in men and arthritis in women. Again, overweight adolescents became overweight adults. Not only are overweight children at risk from physical disorders, they have also been shown to be more prone to emotional disorders than their normal weight peers.

✔ **FACT • Obesity Costs**

Obesity has been found to be more strongly linked to chronic diseases than poverty, smoking, or drinking alcohol. Obese individuals spend more on health care and on medications that non-obese individuals. This applies to children as well. In the United States, hospitalizations among children and adolescents for diseases associated with obesity increased sharply between 1979 and 1999. Related hospital costs more than tripled.

Metabolic Syndrome or Syndrome X

Overweight and obesity are not just problems of too much weight, or even too much body fat. Excess body fat can trigger many abnormalities in the body's metabolism that lead to other risk factors for health problems, such as diabetes, high cholesterol, and high blood pressure. When the metabolism is so disturbed that these other problems happen, we call this the metabolic syndrome. This condition is also called syndrome X or the insulin resistance syndrome.

Perhaps the chief abnormality leading to the metabolic syndrome relates to the hormone insulin and the body's response to it. Insulin is a hormone produced by your pancreas that acts to control the level of blood sugar. If insulin is not present, blood sugar levels can rise uncontrollably and lead to the symptoms and signs of diabetes. Instead of developing low levels of insulin, overweight people can gradually develop a failure to respond or a resistance to the actions of insulin, which can lead to diabetes. This type of diabetes, now called type 2 diabetes, used to be called adult-onset diabetes. However, the condition is no longer an adult-onset disease because more and more overweight children and adolescents are developing it.

Working Terms: Metabolism

Our metabolism can be thought of as the rate in which we use energy to keep our body functioning. Our body uses energy to keep the heart beating and the lungs breathing, to keep us warm, to digest food, and to allow our muscles to work. Our metabolism provides the energy for all these functions. Some people's bodies need to use more energy to perform all necessary functions. These people are said to have a higher metabolism. When people have a higher metabolism, they need to eat more and are less likely to become overweight.

Since diabetes, high cholesterol, and high blood pressure are all major risk factors for heart disease, the development of the metabolic syndrome is a serious health problem. This leads to heart disease at young ages, and now occurs in increasing numbers of overweight children. The Bogalusa Heart Study in the United States, a major study of risk factors for heart disease in children, has shown over time that more and more children are developing the features of the metabolic syndrome, and that this continues into adulthood. This has also been shown in a Canadian study (The Quebec Family Study).

The presence of the metabolic syndrome is directly related to overweight. A United States survey in 2003 estimated that 4% of adolescents aged 12 to 19 years have the metabolic syndrome. It was more common in boys than girls, and increased to 29% in adolescents who were overweight, versus less than 1% of those who were normal weight. They estimated that 910,000 adolescents in the United States had the metabolic syndrome.

Main Features of the Metabolic Syndrome

- Obesity
- Insulin resistance or diabetes
- Abnormal blood cholesterol
- High blood pressure

Glucose Intolerance

Normally, when we eat glucose in the form of sugars, it is absorbed into the circulatory systems. Insulin then acts to trigger the body to clear the sugars from the blood. In people with resistance to insulin, the blood sugars are not cleared and the sugar or glucose level rises in the blood. When this happens, the person is said to have glucose intolerance, which is an early feature of the metabolic syndrome, and puts the person at risk for developing diabetes.

Glucose intolerance has become an important concern for overweight children and adolescents. A study showed that 25% of obese and 21% of overweight children had glucose intolerance, with 4% having undiagnosed diabetes.

Diabetes (Type 2)

As more and more children become overweight and obese, more and more children are developing type 2 diabetes. In the past, the majority of children with diabetes had type 1 diabetes, which is due to a failure of the pancreas to make insulin. A recent study showed that before 1992 only 2% to 4% of children who were diabetics had type 2 diabetes, but that this had increased to 16% by 1994. Obese children and adolescents are also reported to be 12.6 times more likely than non-obese children to have high fasting blood insulin levels, a risk factor for type 2 diabetes.

Diabetics have an increased risk of developing heart disease, stroke, and poor circulation, sometimes leading to limb amputation, as well as damage to smaller arteries, such as in the kidneys, leading to kidney failure, and in the eyes, leading to blindness.

✔ FACT • Type 2 'Childhood' Diabetes

Type 2 diabetes, once almost never seen in adolescents, now accounts for as many as half of all new diagnoses of diabetes in North America. The increase in type 2 diabetes in children represents a serious development, as diabetes is a major risk factor in the development of heart disease, blindness, and kidney failure.

High Blood Pressure (Hypertension)

High blood pressure is a feature of the metabolic syndrome. Recent studies have shown that blood pressure in children and adolescents is getting higher, which is concerning because high blood pressure can be damaging to the arteries of the body, leading to many of the same complications seen in diabetics.

As the heart beats and pushes blood through the circulation system, it creates pressure in the arteries, which rises when the heart squeezes and falls when the heart relaxes. Blood pressure readings are usually reported as two numbers. A normal blood pressure in an adult might be reported as 120/80. The first higher number represents the systolic blood pressure, or the highest pressure in the arteries when the heart is squeezing. The second lower number represents the diastolic blood pressure, or the lowest pressure in the arteries when the heart is relaxing. Either or both the systolic and diastolic pressures may be higher than normal in overweight persons.

✔ FACT • Rising Blood Pressure

High blood pressure levels have been found to occur about 9 times more often among obese children and adolescents (ages 5 to 18 years) than in those who are not obese. A study has shown that overweight children and adolescents are 2.4 times more likely to have high diastolic blood pressure and 4.5 times more likely to have high systolic blood pressure than their non-overweight friends and classmates.

Abnormal Blood Cholesterol

People with the metabolic syndrome can have abnormalities in their blood cholesterol that can lead to damage of their arteries. Cholesterol is transported in the blood packaged in little particles. There are a number of different particles.

The particle called low-density lipoprotein or LDL (sometimes called 'bad' cholesterol) contains the highest strength of cholesterol, and also is the particle that deposits cholesterol into the walls of the arteries. High levels of LDL lead to heart disease and stroke as the arteries get thickened and narrowed.

High-density lipoprotein or HDL (sometimes called 'good' cholesterol) is one of the smallest particles, and acts to remove cholesterol from the walls of the arteries. In the metabolic syndrome, people have low levels of HDL, and the LDL particle becomes smaller and more concentrated, which makes it more likely to be deposited in the walls of the arteries. There is also a high level of triglycerides, which is a form of fat that usually comes from the fat in foods we eat.

✔️ FACT • Elevated Cholesterol

Overweight and obese children can have cholesterol problems. A study has shown that overweight children were 2.4 times more likely to have elevated cholesterol levels, particularly LDL and particles that have a lot of triglyceride in them, with low levels of HDL. A greater amount of body fat deposited within the abdomen (which is often associated with a larger waist size) has been shown in 11- to 15-year-olds to be related to higher levels of LDL and triglycerides. Also, greater body fat in girls aged 10 to 16 years have been shown to be related to lower HDL levels.

Increased Heart Muscle and Thickening (Hypertrophy)

People with the metabolic syndrome, particularly those who develop high blood pressure, can develop thickening of the heart muscle. Being overweight or obese puts a strain on the heart as it has to work harder to pump blood through a larger body. The heart is like any other muscle in the body, in that the harder it has to work, the bigger it gets, like the muscles of bodybuilders. However, the greater and longer the stress on the heart, the more likely it is to fail eventually. Studies have shown that high levels of fat, particularly within the abdomen, are related to greater hypertrophy of the heart and risk of heart failure.

Coronary Artery Calcification

The coronary arteries supply the heart muscle itself with blood. If they are narrowed or blocked with atherosclerosis, it can cause the heart muscle to die, resulting in a heart attack or myocardial infarction. As atherosclerosis develops in the coronary arteries, calcium, as well as cholesterol, gets deposited in the thickened areas (this is called calcification) and can make the arteries stiff and hard, as well as blocked. We can see the amount of calcium in the arteries by doing special X-ray tests known as ultrafast electron-beam computed tomography. The amount of calcium seen in the coronary arteries can tell us approximately how much and how bad the coronary arteries are affected by atherosclerosis. Coronary artery calcification has been shown to relate to risk factors for heart disease in older adults.

Risk Factors for Heart Disease

Obesity is recognized as a prime risk factor for heart disease in children.

- Obesity
- Physical inactivity
- Smoking
- Stress
- High blood pressure
- High cholesterol/ Low HDL cholesterol
- Diabetes
- Family history of heart disease

Constant Inflammation

Inflammation is one of the many ways by which the body responds to injuries. Many risk factors for heart disease act on the arteries by causing a constant state of injury, which leads to a constant state of inflammation. Some features of inflammation may be damaging to the arteries.

The degree of inflammation in the body can be determined by measuring the level of a protein in the blood called C-reactive protein or CRP. High levels of CRP in adults are related to heart disease and its risk factors. In a large study of children in the United States, high CRP levels were found in overweight children. Excess body weight may lead to a state of constant low level of inflammation in children.

Abnormal Blood Clotting

One of the functions of the arteries is to make sure that the blood circulating through them does not clot and block them. Healthy arteries maintain a balance between those factors that increase clotting and those that decrease it. When the arteries are put under the stresses of risk factors, the balance is upset in favor of increasing clotting.

Even early in childhood, excess body weight has been shown to be related to abnormal clotting, which may be a factor in increasing damage to the arteries.

Asthma

While is may be argued whether or not obesity causes asthma, certainly obese children with asthma have more problems. In study of inner-city children with asthma, obese children used more medicine, wheezed more, and made more visits to the emergency room than asthmatic children who were not obese.

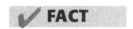 **FACT**

Heart Disease Risk
In the important Muscatine Study, higher risk factors for heart disease seen in children and young adults were shown to be related to a greater amount of coronary artery calcification, particularly in overweight children, and high blood pressure and lower HDL levels in young adults.

✔ **FACT • Asthma Symptoms**

A large study in England and Scotland of 18,218 children aged 4 to 11 years showed that the level of overweight was an important factor related to symptoms of asthma.

Stresses on Bones and Joints

Children's bodies are growing and developing, and their bone and cartilage may not be strong enough to support excess weight. Excess weight can lead to bowing and deformities of leg bones, which is known as Blount's disease. Slipped capital femoral epiphysis is a condition where the top part of the leg bone that fits into the socket of the hip joint becomes damaged, leading to hip problems.

About 30% to 50% of children who develop this rare condition are overweight. For overweight and obese boys and girls there is a mismatch between body weight and bone development during growth; the size and maturity of their bones are low for their body weight.

✔ FACT • Low Bone Mineral Density

Fractures in the bones of the forearm have been shown to occur in severely obese boys. This is related to low bone mineral density, similar to that seen in elderly adults with osteoporosis. Flat feet are common in obese children. These bone and joint problems may limit obese children from participating in physical activity, which can make their obesity worse.

Sleep Apnea

Sleep apnea is a breathing disorder where there are brief interruptions or pauses in breathing during sleep. Since breathing allows the lungs to bring oxygen to the blood, the level of oxygen in the blood may fall, resulting in a decrease in the amount of oxygen being supplied to the brain and body. For the brain, this can lead to decreased learning and memory functions. Sleep apnea has been reported to occur in about 7% of obese children. A study of 2- to 18-year-olds showed that the breathing pattern related to sleep apnea was 4.6 times more common in those children who were obese and had other family members with sleep apnea. Another study of 41 obese children found that one-third had some of the symptoms related to sleep apnea.

Fatty Liver

In overweight and obese people, the liver can become much more fatty. This can interfere with the function of the liver, and in severe cases can lead to liver damage such as cirrhosis, similar to that seen in alcoholics. When the function of the liver becomes abnormal, enzymes made by the liver enter the blood. We can measure the levels of these enzymes. High levels of liver enzymes are often seen in obese children and adolescents. In a large study in Japan, more than 10% of all obese children seen in a general obesity clinic had moderate increases in liver enzymes, and this was frequently related to signs of liver damage.

Gallstones

Gallstones and gallbladder attacks are rare in children. However, they become more common with obesity. A study showed that half of adolescents who had gallbladder attacks were obese.

Rare Conditions

Pseudotumor cerebri is a rare condition where the pressure inside the head increases for no apparent reason, putting pressure on the brain and nerves. The majority of persons who develop this condition are obese. In a study looking at children and adolescents who had developed pseudotumor cerebri, 43% of patients aged 3 to 11 years were obese, 81% aged 12 to 14 years and 91% of those ages 15 to 17 years.

Studies have shown that girls who are overweight start puberty much sooner than non-overweight girls. Certain kidney conditions can be related to severe obesity.

CASE STUDY Anne's Family

How Did This Happen?

Anne never considered before that her son Cody had a weight problem. She had just assumed that he would outgrow it when he went through puberty. He was just a big boy.

Cody had always been a "good eater," although he did not eat a lot of fruits and vegetables, preferring instead more bread and pasta. She had indulged his requests for chips and snack foods, although recently there had been some conflict when she had tried to set some limits. While she thought that he was an active child, he preferred to spend a lot of time either watching television or playing video games. Lately, there had been some teasing at school about his weight, which had upset him, but the teacher seemed to have the situation under control.

Anne had to admit, maybe there was a problem.

continued on page 36

Emotional Well-Being

In addition to the physical problems overweight may cause for young people, it may have an impact on emotional well-being.

Depression

Depression and overweight or obesity in children and adolescents sometimes occur together. It is not known which one is more likely to occur before the other, but certainly obese children are at risk for being depressed. Psychosocial problems during childhood have been shown to increase the later risk of obesity. Children who suffer from parental neglect, depression, or other related psychosocial problems are at greatly increased risk for obesity during childhood and later in life.

However, depression is much more likely to be caused or made worse by obesity. Several studies have found an increased risk of depression among obese children who seek help for their obesity. In addition, increasing depression has been shown to be associated with decreasing self-esteem.

Prejudice

Prejudice and misperceptions regarding obese people are widely held throughout society, even among children, and are formed early in a child's life. In response to drawings, 3-year-olds have described the characteristics of obese persons as mean, stupid, ugly, lazy and having few friends. Preschool children aged 3 to 5 years judged overweight persons to be mean and less desirable as a playmate. Children aged 4 to 11 years have described obese persons as ugly, selfish, lazy, stupid, dishonest, socially isolated, and subject to teasing. One study showed that 9-year-olds associate overweight body shapes with poor health, poor social functioning, and poor school performance.

The problem may be getting worse. A study first performed in 1961 was repeated in 2001. Children in Grades 5 and 6 were asked to rank six drawings of children with obesity, various disabilities, or no disability ('healthy'), in order of how well they liked each child. Children in both the 2001 and the 1961 study liked the drawing of the obese child least. The obese child was liked significantly less in the 2001 study than in 1961. Girls liked the obese child less than boys did,

---

✔ FACT

Feeling the Weight

A study of Grade 3 students reported greater symptoms of depression among overweight girls, and noted that an important contributing factor to depression was a concern about being overweight.

CASE STUDY Ryan's Family

Peer Problems

Ryan was a lively and popular third grader. As the "class clown," Ryan enjoyed being the center of attention. While Miss Henderson, his classroom teacher, was often unimpressed by Ryan's disruptive antics, she described him as "a handful, but a genuinely good kid." When Ryan's eighth birthday invitations went out, a stream of "yes" responses followed, since not only was it Ryan's birthday party, but it was a pool party!

"What's this I hear about a pool party?" The boys turned toward the all too familiar voice of Mark Evans, the ringleader of a small but intimidating group of Grade 4 students. Mark and his friends liked making the third graders squirm. Ryan's friends quickly looked down at their lunches, not wanting to make eye contact with the older boys. Ryan peeped up, "Yeah, I'm having the coolest pool party for my birthday on Saturday. It's going to be so much fun with tons of treats."

"A pool party, eh!" Mark replied. "There won't be any water left after you jump in the pool, Fatty. Bet you look like a whale in a bathing suit. No cannonball contest for sure!" Mark's crew burst into laughter, nudging each other and making faces. "Whale, whale!" one boy started chanting as the others joined in. Even some of Ryan's classmates couldn't help looking at one another and quietly giggling. Ryan's face turned a deep shade of red. Usually his comebacks were quick and sharp, but today he was speechless as he was trying desperately to hold back tears. "Look at your lunch, Fatty," taunted Mark. "Chocolate bars and cheese puffs. No wonder you're huge. I'm surprised you fit in that chair." The crew burst into laughter and once again the chant began, "Whale, whale!"

continued on page 35

and the healthy child was ranked higher in 2001 than in 1961. The difference in rankings between the healthy and obese child was wider in 2001.

Self-Esteem

Overweight children are readily accepting the societal messages that weight is within personal control and they are blaming themselves for the negative social experiences that they must face. Research outside of North America studying 9- to 12-year-old children found that obese children had lower self-perceptions and more negative feelings of self-worth than non-obese children. Obese children with decreasing levels of self-esteem develop higher rates of sadness, loneliness and nervousness, and are more likely to become involved with high-risk behaviors, such as smoking or consuming alcohol.

> ✔ **FACT • Shame and Guilt**
>
> A study of children aged 9 to 11 years found lower levels of self-esteem among overweight children when compared to normal weight peers. Overweight children with the lowest self-esteem believed that they had personally caused their weight problem. These children also felt extremely ashamed about their weight. They felt that this was the main reason for having few friends and being excluded from social activities, with 90% believing that teasing and harassment from peers would stop if they could lose weight and with 69% believing that they would have more friends if they were thinner.

> ✔ **FACT**
>
> **Thin Ideals**
> In a study of Grade 4 children, 49% of girls and 30% of boys chose ideal body sizes thinner than their own, and only 10% of boys and 11% of girls selected a body size larger than their own.

Girls More than Boys

The problem and impact may be greater in girls. A study of 5-year-old girls showed that those who were of higher weight had already developed a negative self-image, and reported a lower body image and felt that they had lower intelligence than girls with normal weight status. Negative self-image was also related to the level of the parents' concern about the child's weight and their use of food restrictions. A study of obese Hispanic and white girls showed lower levels of self-esteem by early adolescence. Another study of 10- to 16-year-olds showed lower body esteem was more common among the overweight girls.

Parental Influence

There is some parental influence on how children view themselves. In a study of 9- to 11-year-old children and their parents, the effect on self-esteem of body size, parental assessment of body size, and the children's beliefs about parental assessment of body size was determined. Children were shown to guess accurately how their parents assessed them. Lower self-esteem was related to how dissatisfied the parents actually were with the child's body size, and the degree to which the child believed that the parents were dissatisfied.

Social Isolation

Many overweight children and adolescents are socially isolated. Such isolation may worsen the social and emotional impact of overweight in this age group. In a large study, overweight adolescents were found to be more socially isolated than their normal weight peers and to be outside of social circles. Although overweight adolescents reported that they had a similar number of friends, they were less likely to be listed as a friend by others compared to their normal weight peers. Overweight adolescents were also more likely to receive no friendship nominations at all. Decreased number of friendship nominations was related to increased television viewing, decreased sports participation, and decreased participation in school clubs.

Teasing and Bullying

In a study of 50 overweight adolescent girls, 96% reported being teased or bullied because of their weight. Peers were the most likely to make harmful comments, and school was the most common place. These girls also reported that they had not yet learned how to cope with these experiences effectively.

In a study to determine the associations of weight-related teasing from peers and family members and body satisfaction, self-esteem, symptoms of depression, and suicidal thinking and attempts, a survey was conducted of 4746 adolescents in Grades 7 to 12 from 31 public middle schools and high schools. Teasing by peers was reported by 30% of girls and 25% of boys; 29% of girls and 16% of boys reporting teasing by family members.

> ✔ **FACT**
>
> **Social Isolation**
> Severe social isolation from peers may have dire consequences. A study has shown that adolescents who reported being teased about their weight were more dissatisfied with their bodies and considered and attempted suicide more often than peers who didn't report being teased.

> ✔ **FACT • No Fun**
>
> Teasing about body weight has been consistently associated with low body satisfaction, low self-esteem, more symptoms of depression, and thinking about and attempting suicide, regardless of the adolescents' actual body weight. These associations were similar for boys and girls, regardless of ethnic and racial background. Furthermore, teasing from both peers and family members was associated with the highest likelihood of emotional health problems.

Parent Pressure

Research has found connections between parental 'concern' about their child's weight and decreased self-esteem, body esteem, and lower expectations regarding both physical and intellectual ability in children as young as 5 years old. In a study of 9- to 11-year-olds, their parents were more likely to describe girls as too heavy and boys as too thin, even though both groups were of average weight. Parental perceptions of overweight resulted in low self-esteem among daughters. Children were keenly aware of their parents' judgments about their bodies. They were able to predict parental responses about their body size with great accuracy. Another study found that children whose parents had greater concern about their child's body size were more likely to distort their perceptions about their child's body as too heavy.

Parents may communicate with their children in ways that give support to stereotypes about obese children. In one study, parents were shown three pictures of children (an average-weight child, an obese child, and a handicapped child) and asked to tell a story about each picture to their own child. Parents represented the obese child as having the most negative self-esteem and self-concept of all three children. There were also important differences among the three types of stories on the chance of successful outcomes or "happy ending" at the end of the story: for the handicapped and the average child, this was 80% and 45%, respectively. However, none of the stories about the obese child had happy endings. This study provides a small look into the way parents may subtly pass on their stereotyped outlook about obese children at home.

Q: Can being overweight affect children's education?

A: Yes, the negative psychological effects of overweight can have an important impact on a child's achievement in school. In a study of children in primary and secondary schools, overweight children in Grades 7 to 9 had lower marks than normal weight children, and were twice as likely to have low marks in mathematics and language. However, for children in Grades 3 to 6 there appeared to be no relationship between marks and overweight.

One study followed adolescents into adulthood and found that overweight adolescents completed less education, were less likely to be married, and were more likely to be living in poverty.

A study examining attitudes toward obesity among junior and senior high-school teachers found important prejudices, including beliefs that obese persons are untidy, more emotional, less likely to succeed and have more family problems. In addition, 43% of teachers strongly agreed that "most people feel uncomfortable when they associate with obese people," 55% agreed that obesity often stems as a form of compensation for lack of love or attention and 28% agreed that "one of the worst things that can happen to a person would be for him/her to become obese."

✔ **FACT • Guilt, Anger, Frustration**

Parents of overweight children have reported being criticized and blamed for their child's obesity. These parents also reported feeling guilty or angry that their expectations regarding their children's weight were not met, and frustrated that they did not know how to help their children.

CASE STUDY Ryan's Family

Fighting Stereotypes

Was he really that fat? Ryan asked himself as he arrived home from school. He made his way to the front hall mirror. Standing there, he studied his reflection. At 4 feet and 6 inches tall, Ryan was considered average in height, though average would not serve as an adequate description of the other dimensions of his physique. He had a round face, exaggerated by a double chin and what grandmothers typically refer to as "chubby cheeks," perfect for pinching. Glancing down, his tummy hung over the waistline of his jeans. Ryan touched his stomach. Even his fingers took on a stumpy, chubby appearance. As he stood there looking at his reflection, he realized for the first time what others saw when they looked his way. That realization made the knots in his stomach squeeze even tighter.

Ryan's mother rushed into the kitchen at about 6:15 p.m. "Kids, I'm home! I have pizza with bacon, ground beef, and extra cheese — your favorite!" she cried. Turning to Ryan, she smiled and added affectionately, "Hey big guy, tonight you and I are going shopping for birthday treats. Remember, you can get anything you want!" Ryan looked over at his mother. "Hey big guy," she had said. Did his mother think he was fat, too?

continued on page 88

Social Pressure

Much of how we view overweight people points toward our underlying belief system. In general, our society values self-discipline and there is a belief that all individuals have equal opportunities and are responsible for their own fate. Over-weight people are therefore seen to lack self-discipline. Overweight children are often blamed for their weight problem, and become victims of discrimination and shame.

Parents, teachers, and other adults who work with children may believe that getting the child to 'take charge' of the situation or responsibility for their problem, often by using negative messages, helps to motivate the child for change. Most children with special medical or physical conditions know that the adults around them are there to help them cope with discrimination and shame. When it comes to obesity, however, the very people who should be protecting children also hold the beliefs that obesity is due to a lack of self-control and psychological problems.

✔ **FACT • Beliefs and Biases**

There is no research showing that experiencing shame and discrimination leads obese persons to achieve greater success at weight loss and improved health. The beliefs and biases held by responsible adults and their peers have an important impact on how obese children view themselves and understand their weight problem. Clearly, changes in attitudes and beliefs are important in helping obese children deal with both their weight problem, but also the psychologic and social consequences.

Health-Care Professionals

While we might expect that health-care professionals would have a better attitude, this has not necessarily been shown to be the case. A recent study found that health-care professionals (including psychologists) who specialize in obesity often used words such as "lazy," "stupid," and "worthless" to describe obese people they came into contact with in their personal and professional lives.

CASE STUDY Anne's Family

A Family Affair

Cody's older brother Mark had always been trim and lean. Then again, he was a jock, playing soccer all summer and hockey all winter. Anne never had to urge Mark to get out of the house. But Anne had always struggled with her weight, especially after her two children were born. She watched what she ate and managed to shed some weight by jogging three or four times a week with a neighbor.

Her husband, Bill, was a different story. He had been a football player in high school, but since then showed little interest in exercise and a lot of interest in junk food. His busy job as a senior sales representative either kept him tied to a desk or traveling away from home. He had developed more than a beer gut, and she worried about him. At his last checkup, his blood pressure was borderline high, and the doctor told him to get into shape or he would have to take medication. His father had his first heart attack at 45, and Bill was his father's son, in every respect.

continued on page 57

Causes of Obesity

The answer to why children are heavier and more likely to be overweight today than ever relates to a very simple equation — they are taking in more calories than they are burning off. In some cases, this may be a problem of overeating; in other cases, this may be a problem of inactivity. Often it is both – overeating and under-exercising. Many characteristics of the child's environment contribute to promoting overweight; some children are worse at coping with 'toxic' nutrition and exercise habits. This ability may be caused in some children by the genes that they inherit from their family, which may make them more likely to eat too much or to fail to burn off the calories as easily as others.

Nutrition

Poor Nutrition

Nutrition is more than just a matter of calories or energy. What we eat and drink not only provides us with calories or fuel, but also the building blocks for our tissues, like bone and muscle, and the chemicals that keep body systems running well. Good nutrition is especially important for children, whose bodies are growing and maturing. A well-balanced diet aims to provide these calories and nutrients in the foods we eat, rather than with pills and tablets. Attention and care must be paid to eating habits, to portion sizes and to providing the opportunity and motivation to make good food and drink choices.

A study of mothers of 5- to 11-year-olds showed that mothers tended to feed themselves in a healthier way than they fed their children, specifically giving their child more sugary and processed foods. However, these mothers stated that they considered convenience, calories, and cost when making nutrition choices for themselves, and believed that they always considered health when choosing for their children. The mothers who were dieting tended to make the least healthy choices for their children.

✔ **FACT**

Knowledge First

Many families lack solid knowledge about good nutrition and good eating habits. This lack of knowledge can lead to choices and behaviors that promote poor nutrition and lead to overweight. Studies have shown that families with poor knowledge about nutrition are more likely to have overweight children. Families who are able interpret information about nutrition on food labels have been shown to make healthier food choices.

Mixed Messages

Children are currently not getting the message about good nutrition. From an early age, children are constantly and powerfully getting a mixed message: 'it's good to eat' and 'it's bad to be fat.' Until around the age of 2 years, the nutrition of children is totally controlled by the child's caregivers. During this time, many caregivers become focused on the amount of food their infant or toddler eats, thinking that the more children eat and the bigger they get, the healthier they are.

✔ **FACT • The Sweet Truth**

Research has shown that children consume significantly more added sugar than recommended. Dietary guidelines recommend no more than 10 teaspoons of added sugar per day for an average diet, but the actual intake in 1994 was 20 teaspoons per day, with regular soft drinks contributing about one-third of the additional sugars. Between 1962 and 2000, data from the United States showed a 22% increase in the proportion of energy we consume in the form of sugars. About 80% of this increase comes from sugared drinks. The current trends toward reduced intake of fats has been replaced by an over intake of sugars or refined and processed carbohydrates (breads, ready-to-eat cereals, potatoes, soft drinks, cakes, cookies, crackers).

New Messages

Once children are over the age of 2 years, they become the direct target of other messages. Advertising designed specifically to tempt and persuade children promote mainly fast food restaurants or highly processed foods. Messages regarding the importance of proper nutrition for health are rare and mainly occur in the classroom. The few hours of nutrition lessons can't possibly compete with the daily exposure to advertising and vending machines that may actually be just outside their classroom doors. More and more fast food restaurants are providing their menu items directly within the schools or building restaurants within steps of the front door.

Selling Sugar by the Pound

The greatest marketing toward children relates to highly sugared foods and drinks. At food stores, children may stand in checkout lines with their parent, staring at dozens of types of candy that are unavailable to them. Advertising during children's television shows urge them to get the latest candy treats. As a result, parents are often faced with children demanding, pleading, and begging. The choice is difficult. If parents provide their children with these foods, they are giving their children lots of additional non-nutritious calories. If they say no, this does not stop the child's desire but may strengthen it, such that when the child is in a situation where there is easy access to these foods, overeating and poor food choices may result. The parents are thus put in a no-win situation.

High Glycemic Index

A diet with lots of carbohydrates and sugars has been shown in research studies to be related to overweight, heart disease, and diabetes. Foods and drinks that have a high amount of simple sugars can have what is called a high glycemic index. This relates to how efficiently and quickly these nutrients are broken down and absorbed into the bloodstream. The body reacts to the levels of sugars in the blood by releasing a number of chemicals and hormones, which help to regulate things.

Eating high glycemic index foods, such as candy and soft drinks, is like adding jet fuel to the blood — they are absorbed quickly and efficiently — which then results in dramatic responses from the body. Low glycemic index foods, such as most vegetables and whole-grain foods, are like burning wood — the energy release is slower and more constant. Wide fluctuations in the hormonal response to high glycemic index foods may increase hunger and lead to overeating in children and adolescents.

Q: **Are low-carb, high-protein diets helpful?**

A: Some recent studies of using a low glycemic index diet in overweight adolescents have shown improvements in their weight and the complications of being overweight. These improvements can also be seen in the low-carb and high-protein diets. Both diets aim to reduce sugary and starchy foods and drinks, but the low glycemic index diet replaces them with more vegetables and whole-grain foods (which are full of other important nutrients). The high protein diet replaces sugary and starchy foods with fat and protein, which is not the diet our bodies were designed to handle. This limits the intake of foods rich in other nutrients and has other health consequences, such as high blood cholesterol. While weight may be lost, good nutrition is sacrificed.

Soft Drinks, Hard on Health

Soft drink consumption has increased in children as a direct result of specific marketing and increased availability. Soft drink manufacturers devote a great deal of effort in creating advertisements that appeal to children and adolescents, who are vulnerable and impressionable consumers. While parents may have some influence over the availability of soft drinks in the home, they cannot control the path of temptation just outside their doors.

In 1999, 2.8 million soft drink vending machines dispensed 25.9 billion drinks in the United States alone. Many of those vending machines have found their way into schools. Schools, work sites, and restaurants often have exclusive-rights contracts with specific soft drink manufacturers. Within the schools, these contracts provide support for schools through sales profits, with some manufacturers directly supporting some school programs. These contracts often have written requirements about the number of vending machines placed and required volume of sales.

Soft drink contracts in schools often require that sales are maximized by increasing consumption by students, either by increasing the number of vending machines placed or by increasing in-school advertising. The schools may become dependent on this support at the expense of the health of their students.

✔ FACT • Turning Soft Drinks into Fat

Children are drowning themselves in a sea of sugar that is causing them to become overweight. From 1965 to 1996, the average daily intake of soft drinks for 11- to 18-year-olds increased by 290% for boys and 230% for girls. Another study has shown that the consumption of soft drinks increased by 131% from 1978 to 1996. Sugar-sweetened drinks lead to taking in excess calories, which leads to weight gain. The body's response to the extra calories taken in as a liquid is different than to those taken in as a solid, which may further lead to weight gain. A study has shown that children who drink soft drinks take in 10% more calories per day than children who do not. These extra calories lead to overweight. Another study of school children showed that for each additional serving of sugar-sweetened drinks, chances of overweight increases by 1.6 times.

Replacing Milk with Soft Drinks

With the increased intake of soft drinks there has been a fall in milk consumption. In the United States, the amount of milk consumed per person each year decreased from 31 gallons in 1970 to 24 gallons in 1997. At the same time, the consumption of soft drinks greatly increased. The decrease in milk consumption due to increased soft drink and juice consumption can put children at risk for calcium deficiency at a critical time when bones are growing and strengthening. This may lead to an increase in osteoporosis in the future. In a study looking at milk consumption of mothers and their 5-year-old daughters, mothers who drank milk more frequently had daughters who drank milk more frequently, and the daughters drank fewer soft drinks. For both mothers and daughters, it was shown that the greater the soft drink consumption, the lower the consumption of milk and the lower the intake of calcium.

✔ FACT • Caffeine Addiction

Many of the sugared drinks consumed, particularly those by teenagers, have high levels of caffeine. A study of children in Grades 7 to 9 showed that higher caffeine intake resulted in disturbances in sleep patterns. Children and adolescents can become addicted to caffeine, showing withdrawal symptoms or difficulty in limiting intake.

Fast-Food Staples

Given the demands of a hectic family lifestyle and a constant flood of advertising, the appeal of the easy access to prepared foods is great. An increasing number of 'fast-food' meals (and between meal snacks) are now consumed within restaurants or delivered to the home. A study has shown that restaurant use had increased 150% between 1977 and 1995, while the percentage of meals and snacks eaten at fast-food restaurants increased 200%. In the late 1970s, children in the United States ate 17% of their meals away from home, and fast foods accounted for 2% of their total intake of calories. In the 1990s, the proportion of meals eaten away from home nearly doubled to 30%, and fast-food consumption increased five-fold, to 10% of total intake of calories. The number and convenience of fast-food restaurants, the relatively low cost for their high calorie meals, and the high-fat content of the foods offered contribute to the problem of overweight.

Foods from away-from-home sources tend to be higher in calories and fat compared with at-home foods. In 1978, both at-home and away-from-home foods provided about 41% of their calories from fat. In 1995, for at-home foods this had fallen to 31%, whereas away-from-home foods remained high at 38%.

High fat is not the only problem. Restaurant and fast-food sources also appear to be a significant source (40%) of the increase in sugar intake seen over the last two decades.

✔ FACT • Not for Kids

While there has been a trend to making available healthier choices in restaurants, these items are not generally marketed to children. While most of these restaurants offered healthful choices on their regular menu, these items were considered only for adults. In fact, the least nutritious items on menus are suggested as the most appropriate for children. A recent study of the food items on children's menus at the top 10 most profitable North American restaurants found that nearly every restaurant mainly offers high-fat items for children, such as fried chicken nuggets, hamburgers, and French fries.

Serving Sizes

Consumers are often looking to get more value for their money, and the food industry has been eager to please. People have come to both desire and expect large portion sizes in restaurants, which encourage overeating and a higher intake of calories and fat. Research shows that portion sizes at restaurants, the size of grocery products and serving sizes in cookbook recipes started increasing in the 1970s, and continue to increase today. This is particularly true for the fast and convenience food industry. As an example, in 1916 Coca Cola was sold in 192-mL or 6.5-oz bottles. In the 1950s, a 295 mL or 10-oz container, and the 355-mL or 12-oz 'king-sized' container were also available, but the 192-mL or 6.5-oz bottle still accounted for 80% of sales. Today, the 591-mL or 20-oz container has replaced the 355-mL or 12-oz container as the standard portion sold from vending machines and at convenience stores. Fast food outlets have marketed 355-mL or 12-oz soft drinks as 'child size,' with small being 16 oz, large 32 oz, and 'supersize' 42 oz.

See More, Eat More

We remember what our parents told us about eating everything on our plate, and that a 'healthy appetite' was a great thing to have. Thus, when faced with a super-sized portion, we eat it. In a study of people of all ages going to a movie, half were given a medium-size and half a large-size container of popcorn. Those who got the bigger portion ate more. Everyone was asked to rate how much they liked the popcorn. Interestingly those who rated the popcorn poorly ate even more than those who rated it highly.

More than just the portion size influences how much we eat. The degree of availability of a food is also an important influence. In a study looking at the consumption of chocolates by women office workers, the amount eaten over the study period was related to its visibility and convenience. The highest consumption occurred when the chocolates were placed on their desks, followed by when the chocolates were placed in their drawer. The least amount was eaten when the chocolates were placed within sight but at two meters from the worker's desk.

Make It Cheap and Easy

Food costs now account for a relatively small proportion of a family's budget, and these costs have decreased from 38% of family income in 1924 to 11% in 1998. Yet pricing can have an important effect on food choices. Increasing the number of nutritious food choices, promoting them, and reducing their cost may be important to changing food choice behavior.

One study of adults attempted to determine if consumption of fruit and salad in a cafeteria setting would increase if the variety of offerings was increased and their price reduced during a 3-week period. During the study time, the number of fruit choices was doubled, salad ingredient selections were increased, and the price of both fruit and salad was reduced by 50%. Fruit and salad purchases increased threefold during the study time. Women and those trying to control their weight were most likely to make these nutritious food choices.

Another study looked at how price influenced purchases of low-fat snacks from vending machines. Sales of low-fat and regular snacks were observed for nine vending machines during a 3-week period during which prices of low-fat snacks were reduced by 50%. While this did not decrease the total number of purchases from the machines, the sales of the low-fat snacks increased by 80% and accounted for 46% of purchases.

✔ **FACT**

Supersized
While portion sizes of everything have increased, the fast-food industry now markets to consumers the choice to 'super-size' their portions for a minimal increase in cost over that charged for a regular serving. This greatly increases the intake of extra calories and promotes overeating. For example, a super-size portion of french fries contains about three times more calories (and fat) than a regular-size order.

✔ **FACT • Solving a Riddle**

In France, people keep relatively thin compared with North Americans, despite regularly eating high fat and 'rich' foods. They also have lower rates of heart disease. This is known as the French paradox. Further study has shown that part of the explanation to this seeming contradiction is that the French eat less than North Americans, with smaller portion sizes sold in comparable restaurants and supermarkets. In a study comparing 11 pairs of similar restaurants in Paris and Philadelphia (including fast-food outlets, pizzerias, ice-cream shops and ethnic restaurants), it was shown that the average portion sizes in Paris were 25% less than in Philadelphia. It was also noted that the French took longer to eat those smaller portions than North Americans. The French apparently eat less and enjoy it more, with better health.

Physical Activity

Good nutrition and the intake of calories gives us the fuel that we need to be physically active. However, when we take in more calories than we are burning off, the excess calories are stored as fat. Good nutrition can be challenging for children and adolescents, but there are also challenges on the other side of the equation as well.

Children are less physically active than ever. This is primarily due to the decline in opportunities to be physically active, combined with the explosion in available sedentary recreation, such as television programming, video games and computer games, and the internet. Increasingly, the term 'couch potato' is being used to describe children and adolescents. While the appeal of these pursuits is increased by direct advertising toward children, parents sometimes use media-based entertainment as a substitute baby-sitter, keeping their children quiet and occupied and within reach.

Sedentary Recreation

The opposite of being active is to be sedentary. This does not mean that we are not doing anything. Sedentary recreation or sedentary 'activity' encompasses those pursuits that require a minimum of physical effort. Increasingly, things that would normally be done in a physically active way are being done in an inactive manner. We take an escalator or elevator when stairs are nearby. We drive shorter and shorter distances that we would normally have walked.

Some degree of inactivity is natural in a child's day. They need to attend school, do homework, and sleep. Some sedentary recreation may be desirable when not pursued to an extreme, such as reading. Likewise, television viewing, playing video or computer games, or 'surfing' the internet, while less desirable, are not harmful when limits are set. However, these types of pursuits are becoming more preferred by children and are replacing opportunities for children to be more physically active.

✔ FACT • Adolescent Inactivity

Several studies have now shown that the amount of time spent by children being physically active has been decreasing, particularly during adolescence. Physical activity levels decline through adolescence, and for girls this is related to race, pregnancy, and cigarette smoking. In one study in the United States, 1213 black girls and 1166 white girls were enrolled and followed from the ages of 9 or 10 years to 18 or 19 years. Activity scores that rated the time spent and amount of effort of physical activity were measured. Over the 10-year study period, activity scores fell by 100% to a score of 0 for black girls, and by 64% for white girls. At age 16, 56% of black girls and 31% of white girls reported no regular physical activity whatsoever. Pregnancy was associated with a decline in activity for black girls and cigarette smoking for white girls. For both black and white girls, the greater the decline in physical activity, the greater was the increase in overweight.

Screen Time

Several studies have looked at the relationship between overweight in children and television viewing. Television viewing is particularly challenging for children, as not only is it a sedentary pursuit, the constant stream of advertising promoting high-fat and high-sugar snacks often leads to the intake of extra calories. Over a long time, children's metabolism can slow and make them further at risk of more overweight.

In a survey of 4036 American children aged 8 to 16 years from 1988 to 1994, 20% were noted to have participated in two or fewer periods of vigorous physical activity per week, with 26% watching 4 or more hours of television per day and 67% watching at least 2 hours. Those who watched the most television had the greatest amount of body fat.

A long-term study that followed children from preschool into adolescence showed that the amount of television watching was directly related to greater increases in measures of body fatness. The effect of television watching on weight was worse if the child was also physically inactive or ate a higher fat diet. In a study of preschoolers, the risk of overweight was shown to increase by 6% for each hour of television watched per day.

If there is a television in the child's bedroom, the risk is even greater.

✔ FACT • TV Weight

One study has estimated that more than 60% of overweight in children aged 10 to 15 years was related to excess television watching. A study that surveyed 9- to 14-year-olds in 1996 and again a year later, showed that girls who gained more weight took in more calories, were less physically active, and had more screen time. For boys, increasing fatness was mainly related to increased screen time. Children who watch television during meals have been shown to eat 6% more meat, 5% more pizza, salty snacks, and soft drinks — and 5% fewer vegetables and fruits. They also consumed twice as much caffeine.

More than Just Entertainment

The link between television watching and overconsumption is great. There is a reason why children watching television are eating more and eating poorly. It is estimated that children will watch on television more than 40,000 advertisements in a year. The majority of these ads are for snack foods high in fat and sugar, which accounts for most of the advertising during the peak hours when children are viewing.

On a Saturday morning, children may see one food ad about every 5 minutes. Children exposed to these advertisements have been shown to develop preferences for higher fat and calorie foods. They are more vulnerable to the persuasiveness of advertising than adults. A study of 2- to 6-year-olds showed that exposure to a 30-second advertisement increased the likelihood that the child would select the advertised foods when they are given a number of choices. Another study has shown that the more a child sees a food advertised on television, the more likely they are to request that food and the more likely parents are to buy it. Ads for foods suggest that the child would be happier if they had the advertised product, and overweight children seem to be more influenced by this message. Brand name food products are often linked to other desirable products, such as toys, games and movies.

Reversing the Trend

Some studies have attempted to reduce screen time in children. One study used a program in the schools for Grade 4 children that aimed at decreasing television, videotape, and video game use. Compared to schools where there was no such program, children were less overweight as a result of decreasing television viewing by about 40%. Another study compared two programs that aimed to treat overweight in 8- to 12-year-old children by diet and behavior changes. However, one program aimed to decrease the amount of sedentary time, while the other aimed to increase the amount of time being physically active. After 2 years, participants in both programs had important decreases in overweight and body fat and had better physical fitness. However, while there was a decrease in the amount of time spent in sedentary recreation that was specifically targeted by the program, children sometimes substituted this time with other sedentary behaviors not targeted in the program.

✔ FACT • Like Parent, Like Child

The activity level of the parents is a strong factor influencing the activity level of their children. A study of overweight and normal weight children showed that inactivity of the parents was a strong predictor of inactivity in their children, both for mothers and fathers. In addition, overweight in the parents was a strong predictor of overweight in their children. Another study has shown that children in families with overweight parents are more likely to prefer and spend more time in sedentary recreation.

Walkability and Safety
The opportunities for physical activity in the neighborhood also influence activity levels. One study looked at a neighborhood environment survey and compared the physical activity and amount of overweight of the residents in two neighborhoods. Adults from neighborhoods with differing 'walkability' were selected to complete a survey on their neighborhood environment. Residents of high-walkability neighborhoods reported higher concentration of housing, a greater variety in the use of space, with more parks and other recreational areas, street layouts that promoted connectedness, better and more appealing appearance, and greater apparent safety.

Safety is an increasing environmental concern that is now limiting children's activity, as the fear of child abduction is becoming widespread and reported with increasing regularity in the daily news. As a result, children are playing outside less and being transported to and from school more.

Economic Consequences

There are economic consequences to inactivity. Studies in Canada have shown that in 1995, it was estimated that 21,000 lives were lost prematurely as a result of inactivity. In 1999, it was estimated that $2.1 billion worth of health-care costs were due to conditions related to inactivity. It was also estimated that if one could reduce the percentage of the population that were inactive by 10%, that this would possibly reduce health-care costs by $150 million per year. It is likely that these costs will continue to rise as our overweight and inactive children grow up to become overweight and inactive adults.

> ✔ **FACT**
>
> **Dire Health Consequences**
> The decrease in physical activity can affect more than just weight. A study has shown that decreased physical activity in overweight children may lead to social withdrawal, poor self-esteem, and more concerns about their body shape, which can lead to behaviors that further worsen overweight.

Q: **Is obesity hereditary?**

A: Obesity tends to run in the family. Children born to mothers who are overweight during pregnancy grow more rapidly and are at increased risk of becoming obese adults. Having an overweight parent is another predictor of becoming an overweight child and adult. A recent Canadian Community Health Survey showed that girls living with one obese parent were nearly six times more likely to be obese themselves. Boys were three times more likely. These findings suggest a role for genetics or heredity, the family environment, and possibly exposures in the womb.

Genetic Inheritance

"My parents made me this way" — this popular excuse for being overweight has some truth in it.

Genes are present in every cell in our bodies and act to control both the body's development and functions. The Human Genome Project has estimated that humans have between 30,000 and 40,000 genes of varying size. Each gene is present as a pair, one inherited from our mother and one from our father, each of whom pass on a copy of one of their pairs. Made up of a compound called DNA, genes act as instructions or templates inside the cells to make molecules called proteins. Most genes are the same in all people, but a small number of genes (less than 1% of the total) are slightly different between people. These small differences contribute to each person's unique physical features.

✔ **FACT • Nature vs. Nurture**

Overweight tends to run in families. One study has shown that overweight children ages 10 to 14 years old who had at least one overweight parent were found to have a 79% likelihood of becoming an overweight adult. However, families share more than just their genes, and some lifestyle habits regarding nutrition and activity tend to be similar among family members. These may be learned rather than passed down. The shared genes and environment within families makes it hard to determine how much an overweight problem is due to inheritance and how much is due to overeating and lack of activity.

Genes and Weight

We are now starting to discover that some genes may control processes in the body that make a person more or less likely to be overweight. Genes may play a role in body fat, helping to determine how much body fat we have, the type of fat, and where it is located on our bodies. Genes may also play a role in the body's metabolism. Everyone burns off calories at a certain rate when they are resting or doing nothing, which is known as the resting metabolic rate. The metabolic rate increases after finishing a meal, during exposure to colder weather, and especially with activity, to burn off even more calories in order to provide the energy to power our activity. A lower metabolism may mean that the body does not burn off calories as easily, and some people may be more likely to store the excess energy as body fat.

Some people may also respond to changes in diet and nutrition and activity differently than others. Genes can influence our appetite and food preferences (for higher fat or sugar). Some genes may contribute to how our muscles are made up and function, which may influence physical activity. All of these things help to control the amount and distribution of body fat we might have.

Too Many Genes

The problem with studying the inheritance of overweight is that many different genes are often responsible. Most of the inherited component of overweight is actually due to a relationship between many genes that may influence many different processes in the body. Only rarely have single gene problems been discovered to be the major cause of overweight in some individuals. Scientists have only discovered just a few of these genes. The discovery of these genes is important. If we can determine what abnormalities these genes cause, then we can design treatments for these abnormalities. However, the current research in this area is still very early. Thus, testing for those genes that we do know about is not widely done and not likely to be useful at this time. Furthermore, because only an extremely small number of cases of overweight are caused by these single gene problems, most cases of overweight would not benefit from treatment.

Twin Studies

Studies of twins can be useful in helping to determine the role of genes and inheritance. Certain twins that form from a single embryo that breaks into two are said to be identical. They are nearly exact copies of one another because their genes are identical. If overweight is caused by genes or inheritance, then identical twins raised in the same or different conditions should both become overweight. If overweight is mainly due to the environment, then identical twins raised in different conditions should differ regarding overweight.

Several such studies of twins have been performed. These studies have shown twins are more alike regarding how they respond to long-term changes in energy balance (calories in versus calories out) than individuals who are not related genetically. Twin pairs more commonly resemble each other in how they respond to energy imbalance, resulting in a similar effect on body fatness and the distribution of that fat. This suggests that someone's metabolism is fixed or constant, and that while changing the energy balance to promote weight loss may cause some people to lose weight, it won't change someone's metabolism.

✔ FACT • Genetic Factors

The differences in metabolism between individuals, which are determined by genes or inheritance, may explain why some people are more prone to become overweight or to have difficulties losing weight than others.

Set Point

While some research suggests that genetic factors may lead to 50% to 70% of overweight problems, it must be remembered that *all* overweight problems are related to an excessive energy intake. Genetics may just mean that some people reach a positive energy balance and exceed their requirements with fewer calories.

Certainly, studies show that changing features of a person's environment can result in weight loss, but not everyone responds to a change in the same way, and some people doing the same things become overweight while others do not. The evidence seems to point to a 'set point' for metabolism, which is genetically determined and therefore not under our control. Because metabolism is typically related to body fatness, our body fatness would also seem to have a set point. However, excess body fatness only occurs when we eat more calories than our metabolism is using. Because metabolism is related to physical activity, if we aren't sufficiently active our metabolism will use even less. The combination of too many calories and not enough activity will put the body well above the set point for body fatness.

✔ FACT • Feed Me, Starve Me

A study looked at 12 pairs of identical twin men and overfed them an extra 1000 calories per day over 100 days. While everyone gained weight, not everyone gained the same amount, although members of each twin pair did gain similar amounts of fat weight and in similar distributions. The amount of variation in fat gained was six times higher between one twin pair and the next than between the two persons in each twin pair. Another study looked at 14 pairs of identical twin overweight women who were put on a very low calorie diet for 28 days. While everyone lost weight, the amount of weight loss and change in body fat was much more similar for members of each pair than between the pairs. These studies show that genetics play an important role in how the body responds to both positive and negative changes in energy balance.

The Family

The family is the major social environment for the child. For young children, caregivers have greater control over food intake and more influence over activity and inactivity. For older children, habits formed within the home environment are acted out with increasing independence, but also increasing influence from the external factors, such as peers. There are many things that happen within the family structure and home environment that may contribute to overweight in children.

Clean Your Plate

Much of a caregiver's parenting skills come from how they themselves were parented. Several expectations that were passed down may contribute to overeating and overweight. "Clean your plate" or "If you don't clean your plate you will not get any dessert" are often heard among caregivers. In a study where parents either fed children in response to hunger or rewarded their children for eating all the food on their plates, the children's ability to adjust their energy intake naturally disappeared and food intake increased in those situations where they were rewarded for eating.

Parents are often concerned that their child is a 'picky' eater, although the child is showing normal growth and development. In the early years, parents equate weight gain with health, both physical and psychological. Parents may desire better than average growth. Parents often use food to comfort their distressed children, or to reward or punish them for behaviors. Grandparents and other caregivers may also be involved in this type of behavior, sometimes in conflict with the desires of the parents. These are some of the behaviours and belief systems that parents have that may contribute to overweight.

 FACT

Parental Interference

In general, young children are naturally able to regulate their own intake in a balanced manner, if allowed to do so. However, parents may unwittingly upset this natural ability. The loss of this self-regulation is a major factor leading to overweight.

Q: **Do children outgrow obesity?**

A: While some parents believe that their children will outgrow obesity, many do not. About 30% of obese children at 3 years of age remain obese into adulthood. Studies clearly show that overweight children often become overweight adults, and often with the problem getting worse instead of better. The younger the age at which a child becomes overweight, the more likely they are to remain overweight into adulthood. This is another myth about overweight that needs to be dispelled.

Restricting Food

Well-meaning parents may attempt to control and restrict their child's access and selection of foods, either in an attempt to promote good nutrition or to treat excessive weight gain. This can have the opposite effect, however.

A study has shown that daughters whose mothers tried to control their food intake tended to eat more when they were placed in situations where they had unlimited access to restricted foods. This led to increased body fatness.

Parents who restricted their own intake were more likely to restrict the intake for their children. Those foods that are restricted tend to be high in fat or sugar, and thus the parents may actually be promoting increased consumption and desire for these foods.

Keeping an Eye Open

Even just watching children eat may influence their food intake. In one study, children were offered a variety of foods under two conditions: told that they were alone and or told that their parents were watching. The children who thought they were alone chose more unhealthful foods and had a higher intake compared to those who knew they were being watched.

Do As I Say, Not As I Do

Children acquire many of their beliefs, habits, and behaviors from observing the behavior of their caregivers. Parents who make no attempt to regulate their own intake yet restrict the intake of their children put their children at a very high risk for abnormal eating habits and overweight.

Parents serve as role models, both good and bad. A study has shown that the fruit and vegetable intake of young girls was directly related to the parent's intake. Young girls with the lowest intake had parents who had little intake themselves yet put great pressure on their girls to consume fruits and vegetables. Children from families with overweight parents tend to have a higher preference for fatty foods, a lower liking for vegetables, and eat greater portion sizes.

The School

After the family, the school is the other major social environment for children — and a strong influence on nutrition and exercise habits.

Meals for Sale

Some meals prepared at home are eaten within the school environment, while others are provided by the schools, often through a food service sponsor. While parents may have some control over the home nutrition environment, they often have no idea of what is being provided in the schools.

School breakfasts often include highly sugared single-serving cereals, while school lunch programs often include high-fat brand-name or franchised fast foods. Many schools now have regular 'pizza lunches' and similar promotions.

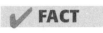 **FACT**

You Can't Have That

One study of young girls showed restricting access to foods can increase the intake of restricted unhealthy foods while also making them feel bad about eating those foods. Studies have suggested that parents need to offer their children nutritious foods and allow them to make their own choices based on their own preferences, without interference or pressure from the parents.

Field trips and school parties often involve fast-food restaurants. Vending machines with high-fat and sugared snacks and drinks are now fixtures within many schools. Packaged snack foods are sold by students in school fundraisers organized by outside businesses that may keep a large portion of the profits. Schools have become increasing dependent on this revenue.

✔ FACT • Selling Poor Nutrition

Advertisements for snack foods and drinks may appear within the school setting. The food industry gains access to schools by marketing its programs and materials to school food service personnel, administrators, teachers, and other professionals. Marketers also access the schools by funding educational programs and by advertisements and articles in professional journals, teacher magazines, and mass media. The food industry may provide food to support nutrition programs or they may provide sponsorship of school programs. Often, this is at a cost of targeting and providing high-fat, high-sugar foods directly to a vulnerable market.

The Decline of Phys Ed

Schools also provide some education regarding healthy lifestyles, either didactically through classes or practically through activities. While gym programs in schools may be the only physical activity that some children get, these programs seem to be decreasing or disappearing.

What Can Be Done?

In spite of all of the data suggesting otherwise, some parents still may not realize that overweight is a serious problem for their children. Many parents view overweight as a sign of a "healthy eater" or a "healthy appetite." They may say of their overweight son that "he is not overweight, he is just big for his age." They may say of their daughter that "she will outgrow it." They may conclude that "we don't care if he is overweight, as long as he is happy."

> ### ✔ FACT • Weighing Health Priorities
>
> Many families have so many other problems that overweight is crowded out. One study asked parents what they believed to be the greatest risk to their children's long-term health. Being overweight was rated lowest of six choices, with illegal drugs being first, followed by violence, smoking, sexually transmitted disease, and alcohol.

Part of the challenge may be that parents also feel hopeless in preventing overweight in their children — and in themselves. Parents do not necessarily believe that their children's health habits are any worse than their own when they were children. A study showed that *only* 27% of parents said their children were eating less nutritiously, and *only* 24% said that their children were less physically active.

Changing these beliefs is a challenge. There is promise, though. A study showed that 61% of parents said that it would be either "not very difficult" or "not at all difficult" to change their eating and/or physical activity patterns if it would help prevent overweight in any of their children. Clearly, overweight is a major and growing health and social concern for children, with many factors contributing to this epidemic. Any strategy or program to help solve this problem must accept the challenge of changing social beliefs, family lifestyles, and personal behavior.

The Healthy Weight Program

There is no one magic bullet that will cure being overweight. Instead, there are many little things you can do to help an overweight child achieve a healthy weight. This book will arm you with reliable information needed to change the eating and exercise habits of your children. The Healthy Weight Program we present will show you how to put this information into action to help an overweight child begin to adopt a healthier lifestyle. It won't happen overnight, but with a healthy lifestyle, your child and the whole family can achieve a healthy weight.

CHAPTER 2

How Do I Know If My Child Is Overweight?

Being overweight can cause challenging health problems for children and adolescents now and in the future. If you suspect your child is overweight, you will, of course, want to help in every way you can. For overweight children who have poor nutrition and activity habits, the sooner they learn healthier habits, the better. The best place to start is by determining if, in fact, your child is overweight or at risk of becoming overweight. If your child is overweight, The Healthy Weight Program can be used as therapy; if your child is at risk, our program will be preventive.

The possible health problems associated with being overweight are certainly foreboding, but we can overcome them with strict attention to good nutrition and physical activity. An overweight child or a child at risk of becoming overweight can achieve a healthy weight. Now let's take a look at some of the ways we use to determine if your child should be considered overweight or at risk of becoming overweight, as well as what a healthy weight might be.

For this chapter in the book, you will need a sharp pencil to record your child's height and weight measurements and to calculate overweight and healthy weight levels in the charts we have provided.

Defining Overweight and Healthy Weight

When we are describing a child's weight, we often try to use terms that will not be perceived as an insult to the child. Because 'fat,' 'chubby,' and 'obese' are often considered ugly words, we try to avoid using them, although with adults, the term 'obese' is a technical term used by health-care professionals to indicate a very unhealthy level of overweight. When adults are considered obese, they are much more likely to develop serious health problems. Applying the term obesity in this sense to children is somewhat inappropriate, though, because their health problems tend to happen only with more extreme amounts of excessive body fat, and may not become obvious until a few years have passed. We probably want to do something about excessive fat long before health problems occur.

Instead, the words we use to describe a child's weight are 'overweight' and 'healthy weight.' However, overweight and healthy weight are also challenging terms to define, especially for children. After all, a gain in weight, like a gain in height, is a normal part of growth and development in children. Every child goes through growth spurts and increased weight gain at various times throughout development, especially during puberty. No two children follow the exact same pattern.

Nevertheless, overweight and healthy weight are useful terms to represent a range of weight. In North America, health-care professionals have decided that children whose level of body fat places them within the top 5% when compared to the body fat levels of healthy children of the same sex and age should be described as 'overweight.' Children with this level of body fat are especially at risk for staying overweight into adulthood and for experiencing health complications.

CASE STUDY Anne's Family

Cody's Follow-Up Appointment

Cody had been quite upset since the last visit to the doctor. The doctor explained that the ultrasound test had confirmed that Cody's liver was enlarged and that he had fatty liver, also known as "nonalcoholic steatohepatitis" or NASH. The key to solving this disorder was to get a healthy weight.

The doctor spoke directly to Cody and was very encouraging. When Anne and Cody walked out of the office, Cody was chanting, "Fruits and vegetables, at least 1 hour of exercise and no more than 1 hour of screen time a day, and no smoking." Anne resolved that she would do everything she could to help Cody get a healthy weight.

continued on page 60

Working Terms: **Overweight and Healthy Weight**

We can define 'overweight' as having a certain amount of excessive body fat that is associated with health problems or medical complications, while 'healthy weight' can be defined as having a body fat level within a normal range that is associated with healthy growth and well-being. These are our working terms.

Put simply, the term overweight means that a person is carrying an excess amount of body fat that is high enough to lead to serious health problems, such as high blood pressure, diabetes, and heart disease. These health problems may result in a need for medications and may shorten life. When people are overweight, they tend to have trouble living a normal life and being physically active, even playing recreational games. They get tired more easily. And they often don't feel as happy as people who are in good physical condition.

There are a number of accepted procedures for measuring the level of fat in a child's body, including growth curves and the body mass index. Parents can use these scales to determine if their children are at a healthy weight or are overweight and at risk for health complications.

Five Facts about Body Weight

1. Body weight is related to body size, but when weight is out of proportion, the excess is usually body fat that increases the risk of health problems.

2. Determining if your child is overweight means finding out if your child's weight is a healthy match for their height or body size.

3. The sooner you help your child eat healthfully and get adequate physical activity, the easier it will be for your child to keep these habits and achieve a healthy weight.

4. Overweight or health problems in other family members can put your child at a greater risk of developing overweight or health problems.

5. For some overweight children, the help of a medical professional will be needed.

Body Weight

Let's step back and begin with some basic information about the composition of the human body. The body is made up of four main types of material that are responsible for creating weight: water, protein, minerals, and fats. Water is stored inside and around all the cells of the body and circulates in the bloodstream. Proteins are constituents of all the cells of the body, especially muscle cells. Minerals (mostly calcium) are stored in the bones. Fat is stored in adipose tissue, primarily around the trunk of the body.

When you weigh your child, you are, therefore, weighing body water, muscle, bone, and fat. From our experience with other children, if we know a child's height, we know approximately how much their water, muscle, bones, and fat together are supposed to weigh. If a child weighs more than what they are supposed to weigh for their height, then the extra weight usually is coming from extra body fat.

The weight of water and bone in a child's body depends mostly on their height and can't be changed much, since it reflects a person's natural size. The weight of the muscle in a child's body depends mostly on their height as well, but can change a little, depending on the level and type of physical activity they do. However, the amount of fat in a child's body can vary a great deal, and depends chiefly on the amount and type of food they eat and their level of physical activity. By improving nutrition and activity levels that affect body fat levels, we can help children to achieve a healthy weight.

 FACT

Water Weight
The largest component of body weight is water, comprising about 70% of the body's weight.

Weight Scale

Another way to describe relative weight levels is to use this metaphor. Imagine a ruler that shows pounds or kilograms instead of inches or centimeters. The lower end of the ruler is colored green, but moving up the scale, as the number of pounds or kilograms gets higher, the green becomes lighter and more yellow. As you move higher still, the yellow becomes more orange and ultimately becomes red.

Green Healthy Level

If you put your child's weight on this scale, being in the green area would indicate that your child is at a healthy weight. Children who are not in the green area will often move farther away from it as they get older, unless they are helped.

Yellow Caution Level

If your child's weight appears higher on the scale and moves toward the more yellow area, it is a warning sign. Perhaps your child is not getting enough activity or eating habits are resulting in excess fat gain. Your child may be at risk for even greater fat accumulation and for becoming overweight. There is no one specific level of overweight that means the child is guaranteed of having a health problem. Children will have different risks of developing weight-related health problems based on just how much extra weight they are carrying, the types of foods they eat, their level of activity, and the occurrence of disease in the family. This means that a child who is lower in the yellow area but has overweight parents with heart disease or diabetes has a higher chance of developing problems, compared with a child who is higher in the yellow area but has healthy weight parents with no heart disease or diabetes.

Red Unhealthy Level

If the weight is higher still, in the red area, your child is considered overweight. The further a child's weight is from the green area, the higher the risk of developing the health problems of overweight.

CASE STUDY Anne's Family

Weighing In

Cody didn't just have some extra weight, he was at an unhealthy weight. To confirm this, Cody's doctor measured his weight and height. At age 11 years, Cody weighed 51.5 kilograms (113 pounds) and was 141 centimeters (55.5 inches) tall. The doctor used these numbers to calculate Cody's body mass index or BMI. It was 25.9. When his doctor plotted this on a BMI chart, it showed that Cody's BMI was well above normal, in the 95th percentile, greater then 95% of children his age and sex. The doctor explained to Cody and his mother that a healthy weight Cody would have a BMI at or below the 85th percentile. Based on this, his ideal weight should be 40.6 kilograms (89 pounds) or below. Anne asked the doctor if she could learn how to make these measurements, and he gladly showed her how.

continued on page 79

Measuring Overweight and Healthy Weight

There are several ways of finding out if your child is overweight. The goal is to determine if your son or daughter is carrying too much body fat for their body size. It must be stressed that any method for determining if a child is overweight is attempting to measure the degree of body 'fatness', not how heavy they are. This degree can be measured using a calculation called body mass index when your child's height and weight are known.

To determine if your child is overweight, you will need a measuring tape, weight scale, and the body mass index tables provided in this book.

Steps for Measuring Height or Stature

The Long and Short of It...

Since children are growing quickly and constantly, you will need to have a way to measure your child's height or stature regularly and exactly. You can use a wall-mounted height ruler that you can hang up permanently or that you can hang in the same exact spot each time you use it. If you don't have a height ruler, you can use a yardstick or tape measure. You may measure height in either inches or centimeters, but make sure you know which you have used. To make the measurements more exact, you will need to follow the same method for measuring each time. Aim to make these measurements and to complete the following Height, Weight, and BMI Chart on a biweekly basis to monitor changes.

Instructions

Child
1. Remove your shoes and socks.
2. Stand up straight with your back against the wall.
3. Look straight ahead.

Parent
1. Record the date and your child's age on the Height, Weight, and BMI Chart.
2. Place a ruler so it sits flat on top of your child's head and mark off the corresponding spot on the chart or wall.

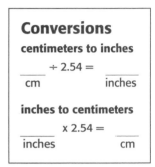

Conversions

centimeters to inches

$$\frac{}{cm} \div 2.54 = \frac{}{inches}$$

inches to centimeters

$$\frac{}{inches} \times 2.54 = \frac{}{cm}$$

Accuracy of Measurements

Measuring in centimeters, use whole numbers

e.g. 141 cm
142 cm
etc.

Measuring in inches, use decimals (.25, .5, .75)

e.g. 55" = 55.0
55¼" = 55.25
55½" = 55.5
55¾" = 55.75

Age Records

Record age in quarter years – 11.25, 11.5, 11.75, 12 years, for example.

3. Either read the height from the mark on the height ruler or use a ruler or tape to measure from the floor to the mark on the wall.
4. Record your child's height in the Height, Weight and BMI Chart in centimeters (metric) or inches (imperial).
5. Mark the date of the measurement directly on the wall or growth chart for a quick visual comparison.
6. Make measurements biweekly (every other week).

Height, Weight, and BMI Chart

Date (Bi-weekly)	Age	Height (Stature)	Weight	BMI	BMI Percentile	Target Weight
Example for Cody	11.25 years	141 cm 55.8 in	51.5 kg 113 lbs	25.9	> 95th	40.6 kg 89 lbs
Your Child						

Steps for Measuring Weight

The Thick and Thin of It...

Since we are using body weight to determine the amount of excess body fat your child is carrying, it is important that you get an exact and correct measure. Every weight scale has a certain level of accuracy. The first choice you will need to make is about whether to buy a digital scale (the one that displays a number) or an analog scale (the one with the dial that spins around). Digital scales will be more expensive but are easier to read and can make it easier to measure smaller changes in body weight. Analog scales are less expensive but will make it harder to see small changes in body weight. Choose one that is a suitable price and suits your needs. You may measure weight in either pounds and ounces or kilograms and grams, but make sure you know which you used. Use the exact same steps every time you measure your child's weight.

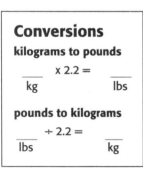

Conversions

kilograms to pounds

___ x 2.2 = ___
kg   lbs

pounds to kilograms

___ ÷ 2.2 = ___
lbs   kg

Instructions

Child

1. Remove your shoes and try to wear similar clothing each time (with empty pockets).
2. Step on to the scale.
3. Try to keep still while being weighed.

Parent

1. Measure your child's weight at the same time of day each time, preferably in the morning because eating food and water throughout the day will add weight.
2. Weigh your child with the same scale located in the exact same place every time.
3. Record your child's weight onto the Height, Weight, and BMI Chart, using imperial or metric units.

Steps for Measuring Body Mass Index (BMI)

BMI Basics

Most people in the medical field, when they study weight to find out someone's level of body fatness and risk of health problems, calculate a number called the body mass index or BMI. This is a measurement of the level of body fat and takes a person's height and weight into account all in one calculation.

The higher your child's BMI is above normal for their age and sex, the greater the amount of body fat being carried. Remember that the more excess body fat that your child is carrying, the greater the chances of health problems, and the greater the chance that your child will become more overweight as an adult.

The BMI curve charts are made by calculating the BMI for a large group of healthy children and then plotting these measurements on graphs separately for boys and girls according to their age. Since all children at the exact same age do not have the exact same height or weight and BMI, these charts have ranges of lines that show the typical measurement and variations around the typical measurement.

The BMI curve charts can give your child's percentile for body fatness. Percentiles tell you how many in the group of children at the same age as your child were higher or lower than your child in body fatness. For example, if your child's BMI is at the 95th percentile, then their body fatness is higher than 95 out of 100 (95%) children who are the same age and sex as your child. Only five of those children would have

---

Accuracy of Measurements

Measuring in kilograms, use ½ kilograms

e.g. 51.5 kg
    52.0 kg
    52.5 kg
    etc.

Measuring in pounds, use whole numbers

e.g. 113
    114
    115
    etc.

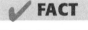 **FACT**

Reliable Risk Indicator

The BMI percentile is the most commonly used measure of overweight and is an accurate indicator of the risk of health problems.

higher body fatness. It would also mean that your child's body fatness is further from the average (the 50th percentile).

You can measure BMI by using a mathematical calculation:

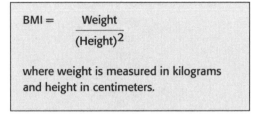

$$BMI = \frac{Weight}{(Height)^2}$$

where weight is measured in kilograms and height in centimeters.

Instructions for Calculating BMI

You can use a calculator to find out your child's BMI by using their height and weight measurements. The formulas to use are as follows:

If you measured height in centimeters and weight in kilograms using a calculator:

_____ ÷	_____ ÷	_____ x	10 000 =	_____
weight (kg)	height (cm)	height (cm)		BMI

Example for Cody

51.5 ÷	141 ÷	141 x	10 000 =	25.9
weight (kg)	height (cm)	height (cm)		BMI

If you measured height in inches and weight in pounds using a calculator:

_____ ÷	_____ ÷	_____ x	703 =	_____
weight (lbs)	height (inches)	height (inches)		BMI

Example for Cody

113 ÷	55.5 ÷	55.5 x	703 =	25.9
weight (lbs)	height (inches)	height (inches)		BMI

Steps for Measuring BMI in Percentile

Now that you have determined your child's BMI, you can also determine if that BMI is healthy or indicates overweight by finding out the percentile.

Instructions

1. Select the correct Body Mass Index-for-Age Percentiles chart for your child's sex and make several photocopies for future calculations.

2. Fill in the table in the upper left hand corner with the information recorded previously in the Height, Weight, and BMI chart.
3. Find your child's age along the scale at the bottom of the chart. Be accurate to the quarter year (11.25, 11.50, 11.75, for example).
4. From that point, move straight up until you find the level of the BMI scale on the left side or the right side of the chart that matches the BMI you recorded on the Height, weight, and BMI chart.
5. Each of the lines on the BMI-for-age percentile chart represents a different percentile. Notice the percentiles are written on the lines (for example, 50th, 75th, 85th, 90th, 95th). Decide where your childs BMI falls:
   - If it is above the line of the 95th percentile, record BMI as: >95th
   - If it is above the line of the 90th but less than the 95th, record BMI as: >90th
   - If it is above the line of the 85th but less then the 90th, record BMI as: >85th
   - If it is on or below the line of the 85th, record BMI as: <85th
6. Record the percentile onto the height, weight, and BMI chart.

Interpreting the BMI Percentile

1. Green Percentile (<85th percentile): If your child's BMI percentile is at the 50th percentile, then half of the children the same age and gender as your child would be fatter (above the curve) and half would be leaner (below the curve). Having a BMI percentile below the 85th percentile can be considered the green area. The higher your child's BMI above the green area, the greater the chance of health problems.
2. Yellow Percentile (85th to 95th percentile): The yellow area for BMI is between the 85th and 95th percentile. Researchers and doctors would consider a child with this BMI percentile as being 'at risk' for being overweight.
3. Red Percentile (>95th percentile): Anywhere at or above the 95th percentile would correspond to the red area and would be considered overweight and at a greater risk for health complications. The more the percentile is above the 95th percentile, the greater the amount of excess body fat, and the greater the chance of health problems.

✔ **FACT**

How accurate is the BMI?

In a few cases where a child is very active in sports, with large muscles and large bones, a higher BMI may be due to a higher muscle weight or bone weight and not excess body fat. This is less likely in children, especially before puberty, because muscle growth is limited. Adolescents and adults who are very muscular can have a higher BMI than is typically considered healthy, even though they are not carrying excess fat.

2 to 20 years: Boys
Body mass index-for-age percentiles

NAME _____

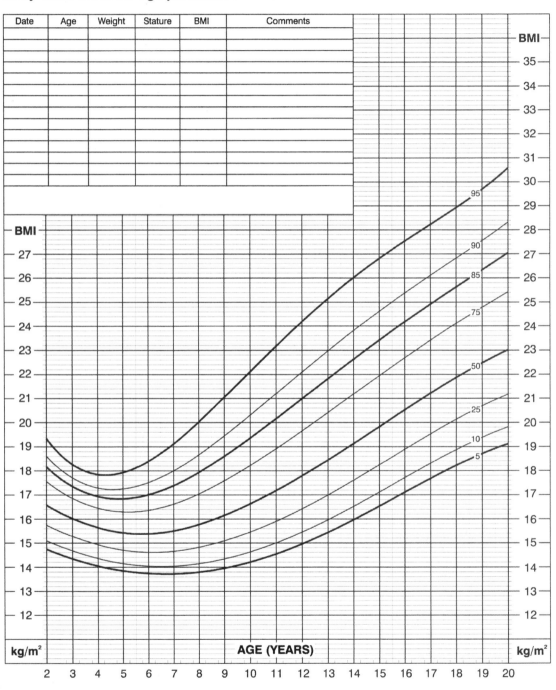

Date	Age	Weight	Stature	BMI	Comments

Published May 30, 2000 (modified 10/16/00).
SOURCE: Developed by the National Center for Health Statistics in collaboration with
the National Center for Chronic Disease Prevention and Health Promotion (2000).
http://www.cdc.gov/growthcharts

SAFER · HEALTHIER · PEOPLE™

2 to 20 years: Girls
Body mass index-for-age percentiles

NAME _____

Date	Age	Weight	Stature	BMI	Comments

BMI

35

34

33

32

31

30

29

28

95

27

90

26

85

25

24

75

23

22

50

21

25

20

10

19

5

18

BMI

27

26

25

24

23

22

21

20

19

18

17

16

15

14

13

12

AGE (YEARS)

kg/m² — kg/m²

2 3 4 5 6 7 8 9 10 11 12 13 14 15 16 17 18 19 20

Published May 30, 2000 (modified 10/16/00).
SOURCE: Developed by the National Center for Health Statistics in collaboration with
the National Center for Chronic Disease Prevention and Health Promotion (2000).
http://www.cdc.gov/growthcharts

CDC

SAFER·HEALTHIER·PEOPLE™

Steps for Determining a Healthy Weight for Your Child

While it is not possible to determine a specific weight that is the most healthy for your child, we can set a healthy range of weight. As your child's weight moves further and further beyond that range, they increase their chance of having health problems.

Instructions

1. On the appropriate Body Mass Index-for-Age Percentiles chart, find your child's age along the bottom scale, then move up until you hit the curve that corresponds to the 85th percentile.
2. Read along the scale on the right to find out what the BMI is that your child should be at or below for their age and gender.
3. Use the BMI at the 85th percentile for their age and a calculator to find your child's current target weight.

> ✔ **FACT**
>
> **Healthy Weight Measure**
>
> The medical field currently believes that a healthy weight represents a BMI percentile at or below the 85th percentile for your child's age and sex.

Determine Target Weight in kilograms:

_____	x	_____	x	_____	÷	10 000	=	_____
85th %ile BMI		height (cm)		height (cm)				Target Weight (kg)

Example for Cody

20.4	x	141	x	141	÷	10 000	=	40.6
85th %ile BMI		height (cm)		height (cm)				Target Weight (kg)

Determine Target Weight in kilograms:

_____	x	_____	x	_____	÷	703	=	_____
85th %ile BMI		height (inches)		height (inches)				Target Weight (lbs)

Example for Cody

20.4	x	55.5	x	55.5	÷	703	=	40.6
85th %ile BMI		height (inches)		height (inches)				Target Weight (lbs)

---

4. Record that weight as your child's target weight in the Height, Weight, and BMI chart.

Variations

As your child grows in height, the healthy weight range changes. For some children who have a lot of growth in height yet to happen, keeping the weight the same or slowing the rate of weight gain will allow them to decrease their BMI

> **Q:** **Does the BMI percentile change with age?**
>
> **A:** Children actively grow, both in height and in weight. As children get older, their BMI also normally increases. That is why you need to use the charts to find out if your child's BMI is similar to that of other children the same age and sex. In general, both boys and girls normally tend to gain more body fat around puberty, more so for girls. This is normal, provided the BMI percentile does not start getting too far above the 85% mark, or, more importantly, above the 95% mark for their age and sex.

percentile into the healthy range eventually. For those children who have grown close to their adult height, lowering the BMI percentile can only happen if the excess weight is lost. This is much harder to do. For this reason, it is better to prevent and manage excess body fat in children while they are still young and growing in height than when they are older.

Calculating Family BMI

A child who is overweight has a greater chance of becoming more overweight as an adult. A child with one overweight or obese parent is at a greater risk of becoming an obese adult. Children with two overweight or obese parents are at an even greater risk still. Both family genes and the family food and activity environment are important factors leading to overweight.

It is hard to help a child with a weight problem when it is also a problem for other family members. A team or family approach is one of the most valuable keys to success. For this reason, it may be important to calculate the BMI for other family members. For other children in the family, the BMI percentile should be charted.

For adults, a BMI between 18 and 24 is considered healthy, a BMI of 25 to 29 is considered overweight, and a BMI of 30 or higher is considered obese. You may discover that other members of your family could benefit from healthier nutrition and more physical activity. A healthy lifestyle is a family affair. Everyone benefits. If you have found that you or your partner are overweight or obese, then it is even more important that you help yourself sooner.

 FACT

Weight Myth

Parents don't always notice that their child is becoming overweight until it is a major problem. They may think that their child is just "big" or that their child will "grow out of it." They may also think that if they try to control their child's weight, it may affect their height. This is not true.

Apples or Pears

All overweight people do not look the same and can have a different fat pattern. The term central obesity is used when the distance around the waist or the waist size is too large. Excess central fat can increase the likelihood of health problems more so than if the excess fat mainly builds up around the hips and thighs. If your child's BMI percentile is increased, then it might be useful to find out if the excess body fat is central.

Fat builds up in two main areas in the body. There is a layer of fat just below the skin of the entire body called subcutaneous fat or peripheral fat. Depending on one's sex, the amount of subcutaneous fat located on different areas of the body is different. This is the layer of fat that provides insulation from the cold and serves as a storage site for energy. The most common place for excess subcutaneous or peripheral fat to build up is around the hips and thighs. This is the most common location for women to put on excess fat. They take on a pear shape.

Another location on the body for fat to build up is inside the belly or abdomen around the internal organs. The fat here is called visceral fat. It protects and cushions the internal organs from damage. Because of the many organs in the abdomen, if a large amount of fat builds up, it can really increase the size or girth of the abdomen. This is the most common place for men to put on excess fat. They take on an apple shape.

Measuring Central Obesity

In addition to determining the BMI percentile, another useful measure of the possible risk of overweight-related health problems is to find out the pattern of the fat buildup, particularly if the pattern is more around the abdomen than the hips. This is called central obesity.

Steps for Measuring Central Obesity (Waist-to-Hip Ratio)

We can determine central obesity by measuring the waist-to-hip ratio. This involves measuring the distance around the waist and the distance around the hips. This ratio can tell us if the abdomen is an unhealthy size and can serve as another indicator for overweight. Healthy waist-to-hip ratio measurements have not yet been determined for children, but as a general rule, the waist size should not be larger than the hip size.

You will need a tape measure (or a string that doesn't stretch and a ruler to measure the length on the string). It does not matter if you measure in inches or centimeters, just a long as both measurements are in the same units.

Instructions

1. Measure the waist size by wrapping the tape measure (or string) around the narrowest area between the belly button and the lower end of the breastbone. Don't pull the tape measure too tight or have it too loose. You should be able to still get two fingers between the skin and the tape measure. Repeat this 3 times. Take the average by adding these 3 numbers and then dividing by 3.

2. Measure hip size by wrapping the tape measure (or string) around the hips where the hips are the largest. Again, don't pull the tape measure too tight or have it too loose. Repeat this 3 times and take the average.

3. Find the ratio by dividing the waist measurement by the hip measurement. A ratio that is more than one indicates a larger waist size than hip size. The greater the ratio, the greater the chance of central obesity.

Q: **How often should my child's weight and BMI be checked?**

A: This is a very important question. It is important for you and your child not to become obsessed with these weight measurements and calculations. They should not be used to blame or shame your child. They should not be used to set unrealistic and unhealthy expectations. Do not get into a negative mindset.

These measurements are only a guide to your child's current state of health, a place to start making plans for better health. They can be a way to set targets and goals, monitor progress, and provide encouragement and feedback. The goal is long-term, so the measurements should be infrequent and non-judgmental.

We recommend checking no more than once every 2 weeks, and less frequently when things are going well. Remember, the goal is to first promote and achieve a healthy lifestyle through good nutrition and physical activity. Much more praise and attention should be directed at your child when they improve nutrition and activity habits than for achieving a specific number on the weight scale.

Other Ways of Measuring Body Fat

There are a few other ways to find out the amount of body fat, but these methods all require special equipment and people who are specially trained to make exact and dependable measurements. These tests are more accurate than weight and height or BMI percentiles for determining the actual amount of body fat. In a few cases where a child is very active in sports, is very muscular, or has large bones, a higher BMI or weight for height may be due to a higher muscle weight or bone weight and not excess body fat. These tests can help determine if the child actually has an excess of body fat or if it is just because of extra muscle or bone weight.

Underwater Weighing

This is the most exact method available to measure body fat, but there are several problems with this method. To measure body fat with this method, the person is placed in a special tank full of water. They go completely underwater, breathing out as much as possible to empty the lungs of air completely, and then hold their breath. The water level and the weight before and after the person is in tank are used in calculations to indicate the amount of body fat.

However, the equipment needed is expensive and not widely available. Because of the underwater procedure, some children are not suited for underwater weighing. In practice, this type of measurement is rarely used for children.

Skinfold Thickness Measurements

The calipers used to measure skinfold thickness lightly pinch the skin and the underlying fat to register a reading on a scale as a measurement of the thickness. The pinching does not hurt. The thicker the skin fold, the more fat that has built up under the skin. The skin folds are commonly measured at the back of the upper arm (triceps), waist, thigh, and upper back.

The person making the measurements needs to be specially trained to use the calipers. This is particularly important if the measurements are to be made for comparisons in the future. Charts and mathematical formulas can be used to find out if these skinfold measurements are abnormal, indicating increased body fat. Most dietitians can make these measurements.

However, this procedure is not commonly used in children because it not very accurate for children who are very overweight.

Bioelectrical Impedance

This is a very simple, quick, and painless technique. Many health clubs and gyms have the necessary equipment to measure bioelectrical impedance. Patches or bands are placed

FACT

Pinch an Inch
There are several places around the body where we can "pinch an inch or two" because of the build up of fat underneath the skin (subcutaneous fat). We can make these measurements more precise and meaningful by using tong-like calipers.

at the wrists and ankles and a meter is used to measure conductivity between the two points from a very light electrical current (a small battery). With these measurements, a mathematical formula is used to approximate the level of body fat, mainly by determining the amount of body water. This procedure is about as accurate as the skinfold procedure.

MRI/CT Scans

Both magnetic resonance imaging (MRI) and computed tomography (CT) scans can give very detailed pictures of 'slices' of the body, showing how much fat is under the skin or around the organs and muscles. These scans are a very good way of determining central obesity. However, these tests require extremely expensive equipment and special technicians and doctors. The CT scan also exposes the person to radiation. These scans have not been shown to be more accurate than underwater weighing.

Determining 'At Risk'

Unfortunately, many of the health problems and weight-related complications that occur with overweight are not easily seen until children are severely overweight. Parents may overlook the signs and symptoms of weight-related health problems, trusting that their child will grow out of being overweight. Doctors can also miss these signs during regular visits. High blood pressure, insulin resistance (which comes before diabetes), and high blood cholesterol are often silent health problems. The only way to discover them is by taking a comprehensive history, measuring blood pressure, and testing the blood, which are not routinely done in children.

Because the health problems associated with overweight are so silent, parents need to be especially conscious of any changes in the level of physical activity of their child, one good sign of a potential health problem. They should also be attuned to any changes in social and emotional behavior. Sometimes abnormal eating behavior and overweight occur because of emotional difficulties or sometimes they cause emotional disorders, such as depression and anxiety. Emotional distress in children can show in various ways. You need to be aware of changes in the behavioral patterns of your child.

> ✔ **FACT**
>
> **Difficult to Understand**
> Children themselves find it difficult to understand weight-related health risks. Unless they are severely overweight and suffering social or psychological consequences, they do not in any way feel sick.

Signs of Overweight Affecting Normal Physical Activity

To help you become aware of some of the clues that overweight is affecting your child's abilities to participate in physical activity, check off any questions to which you can answer "Yes."

☐ Does your child move very slowly from place to place?

☐ Does your child shy away from or avoid most physical activities?

☐ Does your child have difficulty keeping up with friends during physical activity?

☐ Does your child seem to breathe more heavily or get short of breath more easily than their friends during physical activity?

☐ Does your child seem to sweat a lot or more easily than other children during physical activity?

☐ Does your child become extremely flushed or "red in the face" during physical activity?

If you answered yes to any of these questions, it may be a clue that your child's weight is already challenging to them. As your child moves toward a healthier weight and a more active lifestyle, these clues will disappear, even before they reach a healthy weight.

Signs of Overweight Affecting Normal Social and Emotional Behavior

To help you become aware of some of the clues that overweight may be affecting your child's social and emotional behavior, check off any questions to which you can answer "Yes."

☐ Is your child becoming distanced from social activities or from activities once enjoyed?

☐ Has you child been expressing any unusual signs of sadness, anger, or frustration?

☐ Is your child having any problems in interactions with other children?

☐ Have your child's teachers and coaches expressed concern about any changes in your child's behavior.

☐ Is your child having difficulties concentrating at school or while playing sports or games?

☐ Is your child hurting other children?

Any of these situations may be cause for concern and may warrant professional help. If your child is suffering from emotional difficulties, they must be dealt with first before an effective weight management program is started.

Should We Seek Professional Advice?

With increasing awareness of the epidemic of overweight among children, more attention is being paid to the medical and psychological consequences of this health problem. In addition to seeking advice from health-care professionals if your child's BMI percentile or other body fat measures indicate overweight, be sure to take your child to your family doctor or pediatrician if they exhibit any signs of an eating disorder.

✔ FACT • Peace of Mind

Sometimes eating disorders can be confused with overweight problems. For peace of mind and the good health of your child, don't hesitate to see your doctor, especially if your family has a history of weight-related health problems, such as type 2 diabetes, heart disease, heart attacks, stroke, high blood pressure, or high cholesterol.

Eating Disorders

While there has been an epidemic of overweight in children, there has also been an increase in the number of children who develop eating disorders, such as anorexia nervosa, bulimia nervosa, and binge eating disorder. An eating disorder is a very serious psychiatric condition, characterized by an abnormal body image. There is an association between higher BMI and risk of developing eating disorders.

The epidemic of overweight is likely due to an environment that promotes an unhealthy lifestyle, particularly over-consumption of high-fat and high-sugar foods and drinks, together with a decrease in physical activity and an increase in 'screen' time. Eating disorders are becoming more prevalent as our culture exalts a thin body as the ideal body type, leading to a preoccupation with weight and body image.

Children and adolescents who develop eating disorders have abnormal eating attitudes and behaviors aimed at achieving weight loss. They also tend to view themselves as being overweight, when, in fact, they may be extremely thin. They may require professional help.

Some overweight children may also have an underlying eating disorder, particularly bulimia nervosa and binge eating disorder. They may steal or hoard food, purge after meals, and show an abnormal preoccupation with food. Portion sizes and snacking are often excessive. Children and adolescents with these eating disorders feel their eating is out of control and eat what most people would think is an unusually large amount of food. They eat much more quickly than usual during binge episodes and eat until they are so full they are uncomfortable. They eat large amounts of food, even when they are not really hungry, and they eat alone because they're embarrassed about the amount of food they eat. They feel disgusted, depressed, or guilty after overeating. If they are suffering from bulimia nervosa, they may respond to these feelings with purging behavior — self-induced vomiting, use of laxatives and diuretics, food restriction or extreme exercise.

If your child shows any of these behaviors, professional help should be sought immediately. Many children are very careful to hide any signs that they have an eating disorder. An eating disorder is a life-threatening health condition.

Q: **Won't so much attention focussed on the overweight problem lead to more eating disorders as overweight children and adolescents try to lose weight?**

A: There is, in fact, some controversy as to whether attempts to address overweight will lead to an even larger increase in eating disorders. This may be true if unrealistic expectations are held regarding weight loss and inappropriate body image. It is for this reason that the focus in prevention and management of overweight in children should be on developing healthy lifestyle habits, rather than restrictive or fad diets. The focus should be on health, not weight.

The Family Tree

The term 'family history' describes health conditions that have occurred to members of your child's family. Specifically, this relates to the child's grandparents and parents, but may also involve aunts and uncles and brothers and sisters. Some health conditions tend to be inherited or to run in families. In addition, close members of a family tend to have the same health habits and lifestyle. If your family history involves type 2 diabetes, heart disease, heart attacks, stroke, high blood pressure or high cholesterol, then the effects of overweight may be even more harmful for your child. In addition, overweight may cause your child to have some of these conditions even sooner. In particular, if you or the child's grandparents have high cholesterol or you or your parents have had heart attacks or stroke before the age of 55 years, then your children should have their cholesterol levels checked.

The Healthy Weight Program

Although many overweight children are being discovered to have abnormal health findings, the good news is that you can help your child correct these abnormalities. When overweight children begin eating more nutritiously and become more active physically, often the signs of an approaching health condition improve significantly, even though actual weight loss may not have happened. The Healthy Weight Program will help your child to achieve this goal.

CHAPTER 3

Food, Weight, and Health
Part 1: Energy Balance and Building Blocks

Without eating food, we would, of course, die. Without eating nutritious food, we cannot thrive. Food provides us with energy, building blocks for growth, and nutrients to support all body systems.

Without eating enough food, we can suffer from malnutrition and nutrient deficiency diseases. When we eat too much food, we can become overweight and suffer from weight-related diseases.

Five Food Functions

Food serves the body, playing five fundamentals roles in human health:

1. Provision of energy: Food is eaten to provide the body with the proper amount of energy for healthy growth and development. To maintain a healthy weight, the energy intake from food must balance the energy expenditure from body activity. Excess energy from food is stored in the body as fat.

2. Provision of carbohydrate, protein, and fat for making building blocks: The macronutrients in food — carbohydrates, proteins, and fats — are made up of smaller building blocks that the body can use for growth and repair.

3. Provision of vitamins and minerals to support body systems: The micronutrients in food — vitamins and minerals — are critical for every single process that occurs in the body, including bringing oxygen from the lungs to all body cells and converting the food we eat into energy for our body. A lack of vitamins or minerals will eventually cause disease. Some vitamins can only be obtained in proper amounts when fat is present in a meal.

4. Provision of fiber: Fiber in food ensures that it moves through our digestive system easily and helps our body acquire nutrients at a proper pace. Eating foods high in fiber helps prevent overeating and can make us feel satisfied long after a meal has been eaten.

5. Provision of water: Food contributes a large amount of water to our diet, especially higher fiber food, such as fruit and vegetables. Our body requires water to survive.

To achieve a healthy weight and to maintain good health, we need to balance our food energy intake with our energy expenditure. The only way to change our energy intake is to change the amount or type of food we eat. To change our energy expenditure, we need to become more physically active.

In the next few chapters, we'll present the basics of good nutrition and recommendations for changing food energy intake. This is a key means of achieving a healthy weight. We'll then address the other side of the energy balance — physical activity — to show how we can increase energy expenditure.

CASE STUDY Anne's Family

Mother Hubbard's Cupboards

Anne decided it was time to clean out the cupboards and remove the excess of tempting foods. She was surprised to find that at least half of cupboard space was occupied by snack foods, such as chips, cookies, crackers, pretzels, nachos, and granola bars. Tucked way in the back was a very stale package of rice cakes that had never been opened. She had just read an article about trans fats, and was shocked to learn that these shelves were swimming in them. The bottom cupboard was full of the boys' favorite soft drinks and juice boxes. The breakfast cereal selection was up to date with the latest brands advertised on Saturday morning television; Cody always insisted on them.

The refrigerator was full of ready-to-serve entrées and condiments, with a sad head of lettuce, a cucumber, and two withered tomatoes. The freezer was full of pizza snacks, frozen pizzas, and a gallon tub of ice cream. There wasn't a piece of fruit to be found anywhere in the kitchen.

She wondered, "Did I really buy all this stuff?" She decided that instead of throwing everything away, which would result in a family revolt, her plan of attack would be more subtle. From now on, each week she would replace a few items with similar but healthier alternatives.

continued on page 99

Food as an Energy Source

Food provides us with pleasure when we eat it but, more importantly, it provides the energy we need to stay alive. Energy is necessary for every process that happens in the body. Energy is used when our heart squeezes to pump blood around the body, when we breathe, when we use our brain, when we flex our muscles to do work. Energy is also needed to keep the body at a normal temperature — and for digesting the food that is the very source of our energy.

Energy Balance

Energy Balance

Healthy Energy
Food should be eaten to provide the body with the proper amount of energy for healthy growth and development.

Positive Energy
Every time we give our body more food energy than it needs, it stores any extra energy as body fat.

Negative Energy
When our body uses more energy than we provide it from food, the extra energy comes from stored body fat.

For a healthy weight, the amount of energy in the food we eat should be the same amount that our body uses up each day. That means that there is no extra energy left to be stored as body fat.

The brain and the body work together as an energy management system. The brain keeps watch over the amount of energy that the body is using throughout the day. Our 'energy expenditure' is the amount of energy our body uses for keeping us alive and allowing us to go about our daily activities.

Based on the amount of energy expenditure, the brain controls how hungry we are, which is called our 'appetite'. When our energy expenditure goes up because of doing more physical activity, our brain signals us to feel hungry. When we are more hungry, we'll eat more food to replace the energy we have used up.

The amount of energy we get from the food we eat is called 'energy intake'. When we eat food, our brain counts the amount of energy in that food. Once the brain has determined that we have enough energy to match our energy expenditure, we feel full. This is called 'satiety'.

Normally, when our energy management system is working properly, appetite and satiety work together so that our energy intake is similar to our energy expenditure. When they match, the Healthy Energy Rule applies — there is no extra energy available to be stored as fat. If we always follow the Healthy Energy Rule, we will not store excess body fat.

Working Terms:

Energy Intake
The energy our body obtains from the food we eat (this includes drinks).

Energy Expenditure
The energy our body uses up to keep us alive and to allow us to do any activity.

Appetite
The feeling we have when we are hungry.

Satiety
The feeling we have when we have eaten enough.

Energy Rules

Healthy Energy Rule

When the amount of energy from the food we eat is balanced exactly with the amount of energy the body needs to stay alive and carry out activity, our body will maintain the same amount of stored body fat.

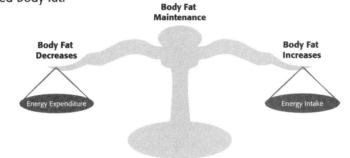

Positive Energy Rule

When the amount of energy from the food we eat is more than the amount of energy the body needs to stay alive and carry out activity, our body will store the extra energy as fat.

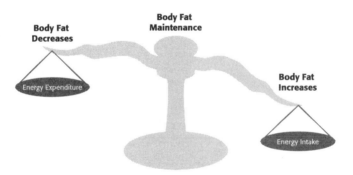

Negative Energy Rule

When the amount of energy our body needs to stay alive and carry out activity is more than the amount of energy we get from the food we eat, our body simply uses up stored fat as its energy source.

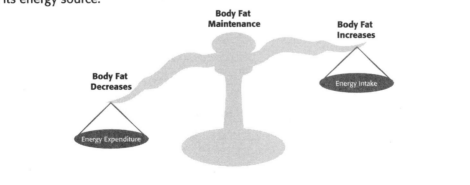

Q: **Why do we overeat?**

A: One reason is that we eat too quickly. Signals from our stomach tell our brain how much energy is in the food we have eaten and how full our stomach is. It can take 20 minutes or longer for all of the signals to reach your brain. When we eat too quickly, our brain may tell us we are full long after we have eaten more than we were really hungry for.

Daily Energy Intake

Our appetite is partly responsible for our daily energy intake because it makes us want to eat. Our appetite can even make us crave some foods more than others. What we actually put in our mouths is, however, under our own control. The amount of our energy intake depends only on the type and amount of food we eat.

The only way to change our energy intake is to change the amount or type of food we eat. The foods we eat vary in their energy because of their ingredients. Almost all foods that give us energy are a combination of the three macronutrients — carbohydrate, fat, and protein — in different amounts. The type and the amounts of these macronutrients in our food can have a significant effect on the amount of energy we get from food and how quickly we reach satiety.

For example, butter is almost entirely made up of the macronutrient fat. A piece of white bread is almost entirely made up of the macronutrient carbohydrate. Two pats of butter contain almost the same amount of energy as one slice of bread, even though their size is quite different.

✔ FACT • Feast or Famine

At one time, food was not so easily obtained as it is now. There were times of feast and times of famine. If people didn't eat enough food during times of feast and store enough body fat, they would not have enough stored energy to survive a famine. Our body takes the safest approach. When food is plentiful, our energy management system encourages an increased energy intake so that our body stores fat so that it is prepared for a famine. There is a problem with this today, however. In the countries where obesity is most common, there are mostly feasts and rarely, if ever, a famine. Some people have an energy management system that encourages higher body fat stores. In others, eating less nutritious foods and having low levels of physical activity can disturb the balance of this system causing increased body fat.

Daily Energy Expenditure

The amount of energy our body uses up each day depends on three important factors:
1. Basal metabolic rate (BMR)
2. Growth and development
3. Physical activity

Basal Metabolic Rate (BMR)

Even when you are sleeping or doing no physical activity, your body still needs energy. The basal metabolic rate (BMR) is the amount of energy your body uses to function at rest to keep the brain working, the heart pumping, and the lungs breathing, as well as for keeping our body at the right temperature. The BMR accounts for around 60% to 70% of our daily energy expenditure.

Factors Affecting Basal Metabolic Rate (BMR)

Several factors we can't control affect the basal metabolic rate:

Genetics: Our family genes largely determine the BMR.

Age: Younger people have a higher BMR. With age, the amount of muscle decreases and so the BMR decreases.

Height: Tall, thin people tend to have a higher BMR.

Growth: Children and pregnant women have a higher BMR.

Fever: Fevers can raise the BMR.

Stress: Stress hormones can raise the BMR.

Environmental Temperature: Both hot and cold climates raise the BMR.

Thyroxin: The thyroid hormone thyroxin is a key BMR regulator; the more thyroxin produced, the higher the BMR.

There are a few ways that we can actually change our BMR. The following are factors that are under our control and can increase or decrease the body's BMR:

Body Composition: People who increase their muscle tissue have higher BMRs.

Fasting or Starvation: Fasting, excessive dieting, and starvation lower the BMR.

Malnutrition: Malnutrition lowers the BMR.

Growth and Development

From infancy to adulthood, the body is growing and developing very rapidly. The cells in the body are dividing, allowing the bones to get longer, the muscles and organs to grow bigger, and the brain to develop. All of these processes require additional energy beyond the BMR.

Q: **How can we increase our daily energy expenditure?**

A: The only way to change our daily energy expenditure is to change one of the three factors that affect it. We cannot control our growth because it is determined by our genes, but we can increase our BMR by a small but important amount by increasing our lean muscle mass with exercise (for example, resistance training). The most effective way of changing our daily energy expenditure is, in fact, through physical activity, which increases the energy we use during the activity *and* increases the energy we use after the activity. Physical activity can also result in increased lean muscle, which raises our BMR.

Physical Activity

Physical activity includes any activity that involves movement of the body. This includes walking, running, and swimming, but also taking out the garbage, doing the dishes, gardening, or any other form of movement. All muscles need energy to flex and move the body. Any time a muscle is being flexed, the energy expenditure of the body increases. Not all physical activities are the same; some require the body to use more energy than others. The amount of energy used in moving muscles depends on the length of time spent in activity, the number of muscles used, how hard the muscles are working, and the person's weight.

Energy Intake and Energy Expenditure Imbalance

If energy intake and energy expenditure are different, then the Healthy Energy Rule is broken and either the Positive Energy Rule or the Negative Energy Rule come into play, with significant consequences for our weight and health.

Positive Energy Consequences

The Positive Energy Rule is the reason why children and adults can become overweight. This rule applies when the amount of energy intake each day is higher than the energy expenditure. This can happen under one or more of the following conditions:

1. Excess energy intake: We can simply increase our energy intake by eating too much food and keep the same energy expenditure by doing the same amount of physical activity. For example, we may continue eating food even when we feel full or we might start eating a big bowl of ice cream every night before bed while maintaining the same amount of daily activity. We might consume extra food and sugary drinks on holidays, at birthday parties, and in restaurants, without increasing physical activity.

2. Reduced energy expenditure: We can eat the same amount of food as always but lower energy expenditure with decreased physical activity. For example, on the weekend we may watch TV for many hours, lowering our physical activity, but maintain the same energy intake by eating the same amount of food we ate daily during the week.

3. Both excess energy intake and reduced energy expenditure: We can increase our energy intake by eating too much food and lower our energy expenditure with decreased physical activity. This pattern of increased eating and decreased activity often occurs during winter months. This combination has the greatest effect on the positive energy rule.

Negative Energy Consequences
The Negative Energy Rule is the key to helping your child achieve a healthy weight. This rule applies when the daily energy expenditure is greater than the energy intake. In this case, the body uses extra body fat as a source of energy. This can happen under the following conditions:

1. Decreased energy intake: We can decrease our energy intake by eating more healthy food (with less energy) and keeping the same energy expenditure by doing the same amount of physical activity. For example, we could limit the amount of foods high in sugar and/or fat and substitute unprocessed foods (fruit, vegetables, whole-grain foods) while keeping the same level of daily activity.

2. Increased energy expenditure: We can eat the same amount of food as always but increase energy expenditure with increased physical activity.

3. Decreased energy intake and increased energy expenditure: We can decrease our energy intake by eating more nutritious foods and increase energy expenditure with more physical activity. For example, we could substitute fruit and vegetable snacks for fried or baked goods and also play outside or exercise an extra 30 minutes each day instead of watching television or playing videogames. This is the most effective strategy for achieving a healthy weight.

 FACT

Food Restriction
Warning! Restricting food intake as a means of losing weight may actually result in a lower BMR and less energy expenditure — the opposite of our goal. When the food restriction ends, the BMR stays low until the weight returns to its original level (if not higher). Also, restriction of food means restriction of nutrients that are important for health.

Q: What are calories?

A: Most people will relate calories to food, but ask the members of your family or several of your friends what they think a calorie is and you're certain to get many different answers — and many of them will be incorrect.

Quite simply, one calorie is a specific amount of energy. More specifically, 1 calorie is the amount of energy to raise the temperature of one gram of water by 1 degree Celsius. We use calories to measure the amount of energy available to our body from the food we eat, the amount of energy the body uses to stay alive (our basal metabolic rate), and the amount of energy used by the muscles to do physical activity.

There are other ways we measure energy; for example, the energy in a battery is measured in electron volts. Different batteries may have different amounts of energy; for example, weaker batteries may give 1.5 volts of energy, like the one in a television remote control. Stronger batteries may give 9 volts, like the one usually inside a smoke detector. Just like different batteries provide different amounts of energy, different foods provide different amounts of energy depending on the amount and type of food.

When you see the number of calories listed on food packages, you should notice that they are listed as 'Cal' (with a capital 'C'), 'Calories' (with a capital 'C'), and sometimes 'kilocalories', or 'Kcal'. They all mean the exact same thing. This is because the foods we eat have hundreds of thousands of calories (little 'c'). For example, a cookie may have 100,000 calories (little 'c'). Instead of working with such big numbers we use the capital 'C', 'K' or 'kilo'. This way we can say that the cookie has 100 Calories instead of 100,000 calories. Just like in the word kilometer (Km), 'kilo' or 'k' simply means one thousand times the amount. Throughout the book, we will use the term 'kcal' because it is the most accurate.

Joules are another way of measuring energy. One kcal is about the same amount of energy as 4 kilojoules. For example, on some food packages you may see that a food has 100 kcal (or they may write 'Cal' or 'Calories') and beside this you may see 420 kilojoules (or they may write 'kJ') .

Counting Calories

Determining the kcal in foods and the kcal required for various physical activities can help give us a sense of how much energy we are getting from our food (energy intake) and how much we are using up through physical activity (energy expenditure).

Counting calories is a strategy used by adults attempting to lose body fat where the goal is to keep calorie intake below a certain level (lower than the number used up by the body each day). Counting exact calories is not a practical strategy for children, however, and may lead to an unhealthy preoccupation with food.

Instead, the calorie content of foods should be used to help ensure that excessive calories are not being consumed in the form of highly processed foods or high-fat foods.

Daily Estimated Calorie Requirements (in Calories) for Boys and Girls

To estimate the number of calories in food needed to sustain children at different ages and at different levels of activity, consult this chart. Use it as a guideline only. If you have concerns about the appropriate calorie intake of your child, consult your physician.

Sedentary children are only involved in 'light' physical activity associated with typical everyday living. Moderately active children are involved in a total of about 1 hour of moderate level physical activities each day in addition to the physical activity associated with everyday life. Active children are involved in a total of about one-half hour of vigorous level physical activities in addition to their moderate level activities and the physical activity associated with everyday life. For more information on these levels of physical activity, see Chapter 7, "Physical Activity, Weight, and Health," as well as Chapter 8, "The Healthy Weight Program."

		ACTIVITY LEVEL		
	Age (years)	Sedentary	Moderately Active	Active
Girls	2-3	1,000	1,000-1,400	1,000-1,400
	4-8	1,200	1,400-1,600	1,400-1,800
	9-13	1,600	1,600-2,000	1,800-2,200
	14-18	1,800	2,000	2,400
Boys	2-3	1,000	1,000-1,400	1,000-1,400
	4-8	1,400	1,400-1,600	1,600-2,000
	9-13	1,800	1,800-2,200	2,000-2,600
	14-18	2,200	2,400-2,800	2,800-3,200

Adapted from the USDA Dietary Guidelines 2005, Chapter 2, Table 3.

Empty Calories

Your child may be eating foods high in calories but low in nutrients. Low-nutrient foods include candy, chocolate, sweetened beverages, french fries, donuts, and other baked goods made with white flour. These foods should contribute no more than 150 to 200 Calories per day for younger children and 250 for teens. Combine these empty calories with a sedentary physical activity level and your child is at risk of becoming overweight.

Nutrient Poor Foods	Calorie Content
Regular chocolate or candy	250
Bag of BBQ chips (75 g)	370
Can of pop/soda (355 ml)	150
Small order fries	200
Large order fries	500

CASE STUDY Ryan's Family

Nutrient Empty Pantry

Ryan and his older brother Dave arrived home from school to a quiet house each day since their mom and dad both worked until 5 p.m. When Ryan got home he usually went straight for the kitchen; he was starving. While his mom emphasized that the boys should choose a fruit as their after-school snack, she was not there to enforce it. There was a stocked, handy pantry, loaded with goodies right next to the fridge.

Ryan opened the pantry door to a world of sugary delights, baked goods, and savory snacks. The pantry contained plenty of sugary foods. It contained cookies of every variety and three boxes of chocolate-covered granola bars. Along with the cookies, sugary cereals filled the middle shelf. The potato chips and nacho chips were kept at the bottom of the panty. There was also a candy shelf filled with goodies, including chocolate covered almonds, sour candies, and mini-chocolate bars. Ryan grabbed some cookies and the chocolate covered almonds, poured himself a glass of milk, and sat down on the couch in the adjoining family room to watch TV.

continued on page 111

Food as Building Blocks

The amount of food energy or calories we eat affects whether there will be energy left over to be stored as body fat. To be sure that the food we eat does not give us more energy than what is required to create healthy energy balance, we need to know how much energy various kinds of foods provide.

Macronutrients

Every living thing needs energy to stay alive. The source of all energy for living things starts with energy from sunlight. The first living things to use this energy are plants. They use the energy from sunlight to make building blocks, called sugars, fatty acids, and amino acids.

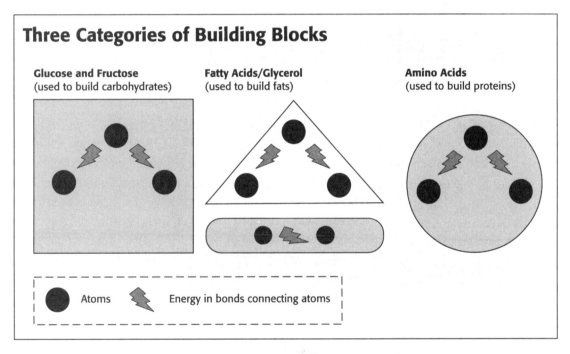

Three Categories of Building Blocks

Glucose and Fructose (used to build carbohydrates)

Fatty Acids/Glycerol (used to build fats)

Amino Acids (used to build proteins)

Atoms   Energy in bonds connecting atoms

Each type of building block is made up of tiny particles (atoms) attached to each other using a bond. Energy from sunlight is used to make each bond. That is where energy is actually stored. The three different kinds of building blocks each have a certain amount of energy because of the bonds.

Plants use these building blocks to build three larger substances or macronutrients — carbohydrates, proteins, and fats. Each macronutrient is made by connecting two or more of each of the three specific types of building blocks.

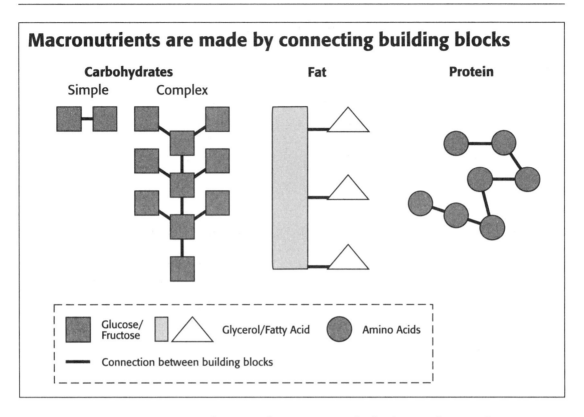

Macronutrients are made by connecting building blocks

Plants and trees use carbohydrates, fats, and proteins to build fruits (mostly carbohydrates and water), vegetables (mostly carbohydrates and water), legumes (mostly carbohydrates, protein, and water), nuts (mostly proteins and fats), seeds (mostly proteins and fats), and grains (mostly carbohydrates).

The macronutrients in these plant products can then be used by animals and humans as a source of energy for growth and maintenance of the body. Animals and humans also break down the macronutrients into their original building blocks to be used for energy and to make new muscle, body fat, and other important tissues.

Three Macronutrients

Our body needs plenty of all three macronutrients to survive. They provide the body with energy and/or the building blocks for growth and development.

- **Carbohydrates:** Made up of building blocks called sugars, carbohydrates are used for short-term energy requirements.
- **Fats:** Made up of building blocks called fatty acids and glycerol, fats help give all the cells in our bodies their structure, serve as an energy storage depot, and provide an energy source for muscles. They are used in the development of our

brain, to insulate nerves, to make hormones and cholesterol for absorption of nutrients from our diet, and to protect our organs. Fats can also be an important source of micronutrients (vitamins).

- **Proteins:** Made up of building blocks called amino acids, proteins are used to build muscles and organs, to make enzymes that help carry out important functions in the cells of the body, and sometimes to provide energy in conditions of starvation or extreme dieting.

Q: **How much of the macronutrients do we need to eat each day?**

A: The amount of the macronutrients needed for good health depends on the amount of energy our body needs each day. The amount of food required for an overweight child will depend on age, gender, current weight, rate of growth, and level of physical activity. We will guide you as to the appropriate amount of food your child will require as part of the program.

Carbohydrates

Carbohydrates are made of sugar building blocks. We get them mostly from plant products, especially fruit, vegetables, legumes, and grains. The type of sugar building blocks and the way different plants put them together make some carbohydrates different than others.

Plants are able to make building blocks from scratch. The main carbohydrate building blocks produced by plants are the sugars called glucose and fructose. When we eat plant products with the building blocks glucose and fructose, the building blocks can pass directly into our bloodstream. Plants also make bigger carbohydrates, such as starches, by joining building blocks together in a chain. Sometimes the terms simple and complex are used to describe the number of glucose and/or fructose building blocks in the carbohydrate and the way that they have been linked together.

Carbohydrates of all types ultimately contribute their building blocks, such as glucose and fructose, to the bloodstream. Glucose is the preferred source of energy for all the cells in our body, especially our brain and all our nerves. Energy from the bonds in glucose is used to provide energy to every cell in our body. If the body's energy needs are met, then excess energy in the form of glucose will be used to make and store body fat.

Simple Carbohydrates

Simple carbohydrate is a term used for food containing sugar building blocks called glucose or fructose or when food contains these sugars linked together in small chains. The simple carbohydrates taste sweet. The chains must be broken back down by enzymes in our gut into single sugars, such as glucose or fructose, before they can pass into our bloodstream for our body to use almost immediately after we eat them.

Monosaccharides: Glucose and fructose are called monosaccharides because they are single sugar building blocks (mono=one, saccharide=sweet).

Disaccharides: Simple carbohydrates with two molecules of glucose or fructose linked together are called disaccharides (di=two, saccharide = sweet).

Complex Carbohydrates

Complex carbohydrate is a term used when simple sugar molecules (like glucose) are linked together into longer and more complex chains. Complex carbohydrates must be broken back down into their basic building blocks, the monosaccharide called glucose, so they can pass into our bloodstream for use.

Polysaccharides: Carbohydrates that have many sugars linked together are called polysaccharides (poly=many, saccharide=sweet).

Starch: A starch is a complex carbohydrate made with varying amounts of two different polysaccharides, called amylose and amylopectin.

Fats

Fats are made of building blocks called fatty acids and glycerol. The glycerol building block is made from glucose (sugar). This is how extra glucose can be converted into fat. The fatty acid building blocks come if many shapes and sizes. The types of fatty acid building blocks in the fat can affect whether the fat is solid or liquid and the function it plays in the body. The first thing to know is that oil is actually just fat that is liquid at room temperature. The building blocks of a fat determine if it is liquid at room temperature. We use the terms saturated fat and unsaturated fat to describe the fatty acids building blocks used to make a particular fat.

Whether unsaturated or saturated, any type of fat provides more than twice as many calories of energy as proteins or carbohydrates and so they are more often a source of excess energy in the diet. If the body's energy needs are exceeded, then excess energy in the fatty acid will be directly stored as body fat. This is especially important to consider when eating high-fat foods.

Some fatty acid building blocks are called essential fatty acids and others are called non-essential fatty acids. We need to get essential fatty acids from food because the body cannot make enough of them. This includes omega-3 and omega-6 fatty acids. Our body can make all the non-essential fatty acids it needs, and, therefore, we don't need to worry how much of these we get from food.

Saturated Fat

Saturated fats are usually solid at room temperature and occur in higher amounts in some meats and in regular fat dairy products. Too much saturated fat is unhealthy for the heart.

Unsaturated Fat

Unsaturated fats are liquid at room temperature (oils) and come mostly from plant products. Unsaturated fats occur in higher amounts in fish, whole grains, nuts, seeds, and some vegetables, such as olives and avocados. Unsaturated fats are considered healthier for the heart. Unsaturated fat exists as mono-unsaturated fat or poly-unsaturated fat depending on which fatty acids building blocks are used to make them.

Proteins

Proteins are made of chains of building blocks called amino acids. The proteins help give structure to our cells and they are also the main component of all the muscles, organs, and enzymes in the body. Most people living in North America get more than enough protein in their diet.

The amino acid building blocks of protein are either called essential or non-essential, just like the fatty acids of fat. The essential amino acids are the ones that our body cannot make enough of itself, so we need to get them from the proteins in the foods we eat. The human body can make any of the non-essential amino acids out of the other amino acids in the body.

Q: **Are all sources of protein the same?**

A: Protein in our diet can come from both animal and plant sources. The proteins that come from animal sources, such as meat, fish, dairy and eggs, are called complete proteins because they often contain all the essential amino acids. The plant sources are often low in or missing certain essential amino acids. This means that when a diet is strictly vegetarian, it is very important to combine a wide variety of plant foods in the diet to ensure an adequate amount of protein and to ensure that all the essential amino acids are obtained.

Macronutrient Digestion

The foods we eat are a combination of some or all of the macronutrients — carbohydrate, fat, and protein — and water. These macronutrients must be broken down into their basic building blocks so that they are small enough to move from our digestive system into our bloodstream. The breakdown begins when we chew our food into smaller bits and continues in our stomach and intestines, where food is further broken down by enzymes. The building blocks are then taken into our bloodstream and sent around the body to be used for energy, growth, and development.

The speed at which enzymes can 'chop up' the connections is different for the three macronutrients, with carbohydrates being the quickest to chop, fats being intermediate and proteins being the slowest. This means that the building blocks of carbohydrates (mainly glucose) are available in our bloodstream first and can be used more quickly for energy. This is why we sometimes crave sweets when we are tired. Fatty acid building blocks enter our bloodstream a little later and amino acid building blocks, a little later still.

✔ FACT

Food Choppers
When we eat food, enzymes in the stomach 'chop up' the connections between the building blocks of carbohydrates, fats, and proteins. These building blocks are glucose, frustose, fatty acids, glycerol, and amino acids. They are small enough to be taken from our digestive system into our bloodstream so that our whole body can use them.

Animal Use of Macronutrients

For many animals, plant products are the only foods they eat. These animals are called herbivores. Because animals cannot get their energy directly from the sun, herbivores get all the energy they need from the macronutrients in plant products. When the plant products are eaten, the macronutrients they contain are broken back down into their building blocks. The building blocks can then be used to build new macronutrients or they can be used as a source of energy.

Usually, the protein building blocks from the plant products are used to build new proteins, like muscle in the animal.

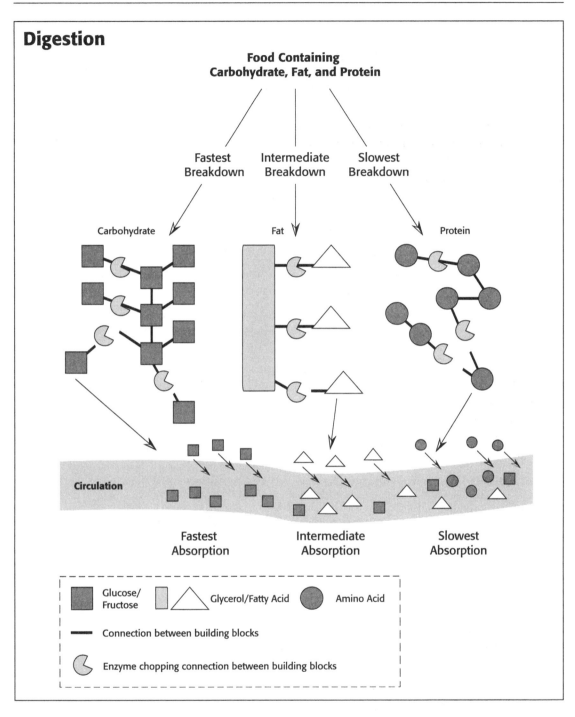

Digestion

Food Containing Carbohydrate, Fat, and Protein

Fastest Breakdown — Intermediate Breakdown — Slowest Breakdown

Carbohydrate   Fat   Protein

Circulation

Fastest Absorption   Intermediate Absorption   Slowest Absorption

| Glucose/Fructose | Glycerol/Fatty Acid | Amino Acid |

Connection between building blocks

Enzyme chopping connection between building blocks

The fat building blocks from the plant products are used to make new fats in the animal and they are also a great source of energy. The carbohydrate building blocks from the plant products are mostly used as a quick source of energy.

Animals use the proteins from the plant products to make their muscles and the fats from plant products to make their own new fats.

Human Use of Macronutrients

Humans are omnivores. We have the ability to get our energy from both plant products and other animals. When we eat plant products, we use the macronutrients in the same way as the herbivore animals. In addition, we can also use the macronutrients from animal sources of food. When we eat animal products, the macronutrients we are eating are mostly protein and fat.

- Protein macronutrients are used mostly to build new proteins in our body, such as our muscles.
- Fat macronutrients are used as a structural component in every cell in our body, as a very good source of energy, and as a storage form of energy.
- Carbohydrate macronutrients are used for energy.

Remember that fats and carbohydrates are made up of different building blocks. When the bonds in these building blocks are broken, they release the energy that was originally stored there by plants. The source of all of our energy comes from breaking down the bonds in the building blocks of macronutrients.

Calorie Content of Macronutrients

When we measure the number of calories in our food, we are measuring the number of calories stored in the bonds of the building blocks of the macronutrients. The number of calories stored in the chemical bonds of the macronutrients is the amount of energy our body can obtain from them when we eat them.

- Fat: each gram of fat contains almost 9 Calories of energy
- Carbohydrate: each gram of carbohydrate contains 4 Calories of energy.
- Protein: each gram of protein contains 4 Calories of energy

It makes sense that our body stores extra calories as fat because, gram for gram, we can store more energy without as much an increase in weight. To illustrate this, suppose we had an excess of 3500 Calories in energy intake. Consider that 3500 Calories is the amount of energy in 1 pound of fat. To store this excess energy, the body will produce approximately 1 pound of fat. If the body were to store it as carbohydrate or protein, it would have to add 2 pounds to our weight, which is less efficient. Any extra energy from protein and carbohydrate will always be converted to body fat for storage.

 FACT

Gram for Gram

One gram of fat can give us more than twice the amount of energy as one gram of either carbohydrate or protein.

Storing Energy as Fat

While plants can store energy in all three macronutrients, animals and humans store almost all excess energy as fat. Sometimes the amount of energy in the macronutrients we eat is much greater than what our body needs. When there is excess energy available from the foods eaten by an animal or human, it can be stored for later use. This is the basis of the positive energy rule. This is extremely important for survival when food is scarce or when extra energy is needed. The body can use stored fat to get needed energy. This is the basis of the negative energy rule.

Energy Intake Variation

We are even suited for larger variation of energy intake and over longer periods of time. For example, when young children are sick for several weeks, their body weight may fall sharply, but upon recovery, their appetite returns, they eat extra, and they spring back quickly to their original weight and carry on developing normally.

The body prepares for variation by building up stores of energy. In times of lower food intake, it simply uses its stored body fat for energy. We do not have to monitor every single bite of food we eat and calculate how many calories and nutrients each bite contains. Our body knows all of this and adjusts just fine.

Vitamins and Minerals

Our body also stores micronutrients (vitamins and minerals) in case we lack them in our diet at some point. Some of these micronutrients are stored in our body in large enough amounts that we can go months without them if absolutely necessary. As long as the foods eaten provide a wide variety of micronutrients, the body will pick and choose the appropriate amounts needed to maintain health and store a backup supply.

The role micronutrients play in achieving a healthy weight is a subject of the next chapter.

 FACT

Coping with Food Variations
People eat different foods each day. Even the amount of food varies from day to day. The body expects this and copes easily with this daily variation. As long as the amount of food eaten doesn't exceed the energy needs of the body on a regular basis, the body will not accumulate unhealthy levels of fat.

CHAPTER 4

Food, Weight, and Health
Part 2: Systems Support and Energy Density

Food provides the body with energy to maintain the basal metabolic rate and to enable physical activity, as well as the building blocks or macronutrients needed for growth and repair. Food also provides the body with vitamins, minerals, and other micronutrients to support all body systems, as well as fiber needed for good digestion.

Eating micronutrient-rich foods will help to ensure overall good health, while eating foods high in fiber helps the body acquire nutrients at the proper pace and prevent overeating. This is essential for achieving a healthy body weight.

Food to Support Body Systems

Micronutrients play an essential role in the body. They are important for growth and development, metabolism, and protection against disease. Micronutrients include vitamins, minerals, and phytochemicals.

A diet with a variety of whole, fresh foods, such as fruit, vegetables, legumes, whole grains, and meat products, will usually provide healthy people with all of the vitamins and minerals needed. Processing of certain foods can destroy vitamins, so some of these processed foods are consequently 'fortified' with man-made vitamins.

Vitamins

There are many dictionary definitions of vitamins that are more complex than necessary for understanding their role. A vitamin is a substance needed by our body in specific amounts to keep our cells running properly. Vitamins are made by plants, animals and bacteria. Each type of vitamin plays a slightly different yet vital role. A lack of any one vitamin in the diet will lead to less than optimal health or even specific diseases. Vitamins are classified as either fat-soluble or water-soluble.

Fat-soluble Vitamins

These micronutrients dissolve in fat and accumulate in the fat of plant and animal products. When we eat plant and animal products that contain fat, we are also eating the vitamins that have accumulated there. The fat-soluble vitamins we get from food are dissolved and stored in our liver and within body fat. We don't need to worry if on some days we get a little less of these vitamins than is recommended because our liver provides a backup supply. This supply can often last months. However, we do need to be concerned about getting too much of these vitamins since they are fat soluble and can accumulate in our body. Getting too much of these vitamins is not a concern when a variety of food is consumed. The risk of overdosing on specific vitamins is more serious if high dose vitamin pills are being used. This does not include children's multivitamins taken as directed.

Water-soluble Vitamins

These micronutrients for the most part are not stored in our body because the water in our body is constantly being recycled. It is more important that we get the water-soluble vitamins on a more regular basis than the fat-soluble vitamins.

CASE STUDY Anne's Family

Couch Potatoes

It was a typical Sunday afternoon. Anne had just finished her jog. She looked into the living room. Stretched out on the sofa were Cody, Mark, and Bill watching the football game on television. She had already made them one platter of nachos, complete with extra cheese and sour cream. Bill asked for another platter and another round of drinks for the "boys" — a beer for himself and sodas for Cody and Mark. Anne looked at them and sighed. She also noticed the couch was starting to sag in the middle.

Anne decided she would try something different. She sliced up some carrots, celery, red and green peppers, and broccoli, and mixed up a yogurt dip her friend had told her about. She made a pitcher of lemon iced tea, sweetened with a sugar substitute, and brought the tray into the living room. As she set the tray on the coffee table, the cheering on the sofa stopped. Clearly this waitress had gotten the order wrong. As the revolt of the couch potatoes was gearing up, Anne stared them all down. It was the start of a new day.

continued on page 105

Fat-soluble Vitamins		
Vitamin	**Function**	**Source**
Vitamin A	Promotes growth and repair of body tissue, healthy eyes, good night vision, and a strong immune system	Carrots, sweet potatoes, spinach and other leafy green veggies, yellow squash, peaches and apricots all provide beta and other carotenes used to make vitamin A. Non-fruit and vegetable sources include liver and fish oils, whole and fortified milk, and eggs
Vitamin D	Allows the body to use calcium and phosphorus and thus important for bone growth and strength, and for strong teeth	While the body can make all the vitamin D it needs from sunlight, fears that ultraviolet ray exposure may cause cancer have caused us avoid direct sunlight. More time spent indoors during winter also decreases exposure. Natural sources include egg yolks and fatty fish, like cod, herring, and mackerel Some foods have been fortified with vitamin D, especially milk
Vitamin E	Antioxidant properties protect cells from damage Necessary for making our blood Helps our bodies use oxygen and protects lungs from air pollution	Carrots, celery, green leafy vegetables, apples, vegetable oils, peanuts, seeds (such as sunflower), nuts (such as almonds), wheat germ, seafood
Vitamin K	Helps our body produce new proteins Helps stop bleeding when we are injured or when we have surgery	The natural bacteria in the gut is a significant source of this vitamin. In addition, it is found in vegetables, such as green beans and green leafy vegetables, fruit, whole grains, dairy products, eggs, meat, poultry, and plant oils

Water-soluble Vitamins		
Vitamin	**Function**	**Source**
B-Complex Vitamins	See specific function below	See specific source below
Vitamin B-1 (thiamine)	Helps convert food into energy in the body Helps our nerves work properly Important for growth and keeping muscles active	Dried beans, seeds, nuts, whole grains, and pork

Vitamin	Function	Source
Vitamin B-2 (Riboflavin)	Helps convert food into energy Helps keep red blood cells healthy Helps our body make hormones	Green vegetables, such as broccoli, turnips, asparagus, and spinach, dairy products, meats, poultry, and whole grains
Vitamin B-3 (Niacin)	Helps our body convert food into energy Important for a healthy digestive system Helps our blood circulation Important for nerve function	Beans, peas, poultry, fish, and whole grains
Vitamin B-5 (Pantothenic Acid)	Helps convert food into energy Necessary to make important hormones, vitamin D, and red blood cells	Found in almost all foods
Vitamin B-6 (Pyridoxine)	Helps convert food into energy Keeps our red blood cells healthy Important for our immune system and nerve function	Poultry, fish, pork, eggs, and whole grains
Vitamin B-12 (Cobalamin)	Helps convert food into energy Keeps our red blood cells healthy Helps maintain our nervous system and immune system	Beef, fish, poultry, eggs, and dairy products
Vitamin C	Important for healing wounds, keeping blood vessels strong, keeping gums healthy, keeping teeth and bones strong, and keeping skin healthy May also boost our immune system Antioxidant	Citrus fruits, strawberries, kiwi, guava, tomatoes, collard and mustard greens, broccoli, spinach, parsley, green and red peppers, and potatoes
Folic Acid	Important for helping cells grow and divide Reduces risk of certain birth defects Important for our red blood cells and crucial in creating amino acids, the building blocks of proteins in the body	Green leafy vegetables, dried beans, oranges, nuts, poultry, liver, and fortified cereals
Biotin	Important for obtaining energy from fats, proteins, and carbohydrates	Spinach, cauliflower, mushrooms, beef, chicken, salmon, eggs, and cheese

Minerals

Minerals are elements that our body must have in specific amounts to keep all the cells working properly. Minerals are not made by animals or plants but are found in the soil. Plants absorb the minerals, which are then passed to animals and to us when we eat plant and animal products. If minerals are lacking in the diet, various health problems can develop. Each different type of mineral plays a slightly different and vital role in our body.

A diet with a variety of whole, fresh foods, such as fruit, vegetables, legumes, and whole grains, usually provides all of the minerals we need. Many processed foods are also fortified with minerals.

Common Minerals		
Mineral	**Function**	**Source**
Calcium	Important for bones, teeth, muscle tissue, for regulating the heart, muscles, and nervous system, and for preventing bleeding	Green leafy vegetables, such as broccoli, kale and collards, almonds, dairy products, calcium-fortified orange juice or soy milk, salmon with bones
Chromium	Helps control the function of enzymes in the body	Peas, beans, meat, whole grains, cheese, blackstrap molasses
Copper	Important for the formation of red blood cells, pigment (which gives our hair color), and bone health	Nuts, cocoa, black pepper, and blackstrap molasses
Fluoride	Helps strengthen teeth	Present in high amounts in many toothpaste brands (avoid swallowing), tea, and the bones of fish. Added to tap water in certain areas.
Iodine	Necessary for making the thyroid hormones that control energy expenditure	Present in milk, bread, lobster, and shrimp. Added to most salt in North America (iodized salt)
Iron	Extremely important for red blood cells to take oxygen from the air we breathe and deliver it to all the cells in our body. Without enough iron, we feel tired.	Green leafy vegetables, meat, fish, poultry, eggs, and whole grains
Magnesium	Important for the enzymes, for nerve and muscle function, and for bone growth	Leafy greens, nuts, beans, legumes, meats, and whole grains

Mineral	Function	Source
Manganese	Essential for reproductive function, physical growth, normal formation of bones and cartilage, and normal brain function	Fruit, vegetables, whole grains, and tea
Molybdenum	Helps enzymes Helps convert food to energy	Spinach, lima beans, milk, and whole grains
Phosphorus	Used to build muscles, bones, and teeth Involved in almost all the energy requiring functions in the body	Nuts, seeds, whole grains, meat, poultry, fish, and eggs
Potassium	Helps regulate blood pressure Important for heart, muscle, and nerve function	Most raw vegetables, bananas, citrus fruits, sunflower seeds, and molasses
Selenium	Works together with vitamin E as an antioxidant to clean up toxins in the body	Brazil nuts, whole grains, lobster, clams, crabs, and oysters
Sodium	Important for regulating the amount of fluids in and around the cells Helps flex muscles Important for nerve function	Table salt and processed foods often provide us with much more than we actually need
Zinc	Essential for normal growth, development, and immune system regulations Helps maintain skin, hair, and bones Keeps reproductive organs functioning Important for sense of taste, smell, and night vision	Whole grains, beef, poultry, liver, oysters, eggs, and dairy products

Q: When are supplements needed?

A: There are times when supplements are useful. Certain health conditions may require additional nutrients; for example, children with extremely poor appetites or who are very picky eaters (not likely to be an overweight child), children with serious digestive disorders (for example, Crohn's disease or ulcerative colitis), and vegans (vegetarians who consume no animal products whatsoever).

Q: **Does my child need a multivitamin?**

A: Multi-vitamins provide select vitamins and minerals in a concentrated form but not the diversity of compounds that occur naturally in foods. Encouraging children to increase fruit, vegetable, and whole grain consumption is the best strategy for ensuring they get the benefit of the vitamins and phytochemicals in these foods. There is evidence of the beneficial effect of a diet rich in fruit and vegetables. There isn't evidence that all vitamin supplements are beneficial. The beneficial effect of a diet rich in whole fruit and vegetables is most likely because the vitamins and phytochemicals work together as a team, helping our body to stay healthy. During the winter, if the availability of fresh produce is limited, you might consider giving your child a multivitamin as 'insurance'.

Phytochemicals

Phytochemicals (phyto=plant) are nonnutritive chemicals that come from plants. They are called nonnutritive because they have not yet been classified officially as nutrients. Research is being done to determine the specific types, levels, and food sources of phytochemicals that are important for health. Once these details are worked out, they can officially be classified as nutrients.

Many phytochemicals have already been shown to have properties that aid in the prevention of cardiovascular disease, high blood pressure, diabetes, and cancer. Almost 1000 different phytochemicals have been identified as components of food, and many more phytochemicals continue to be discovered today. One serving of vegetables may have more than 100 different phytochemicals.

Although it is not yet possible to give the specific type and amount of the various phytochemicals necessary for health, there are guidelines. Both the American and Canadian health and nutrition agencies strongly recommend that we consume a wide variety of fruits, vegetables, and whole grains to make sure we get a wide range of the phytochemicals.

Food as Fiber

Fiber is any part of food that we can't digest. That means fiber in the foods we eat does not contribute any energy. Fiber is mainly carbohydrate that our bodies cannot digest because we

CASE STUDY Anne's Family

A Family Meeting

The family sat around the evening dinner table, and Anne called the meeting to order. She really did not have an agenda, but thought she would first set out the facts and see what response she might get. That afternoon she had talked for an hour with Bill about Cody's cholesterol and weight problems. She also expressed concern for Bill, and how his lack of concern was not helping either Cody or himself. Bill had to admit he was guilty and did not really know what to do, but would follow Anne's lead as to a plan. Having dad on board was going to be critical to getting some change.

Anne outlined how the family's eating and television habits were causing health problems, and while Cody needed some help the most, everyone would benefit. Cody started to get tearful, but Anne assured him that he was not being singled out. Everyone was going to learn and live a healthier lifestyle. She also assured them that this was not going to be painful, that no one was going on a diet, and that everyone had a part to play. They would start out slow and take lots of small steps.

At the end of Anne's talk, everyone was feeling really positive, and Cody decided that they should celebrate with a big bowl of ice cream. Anne smiled — and asked Cody if he could think of a better treat that might be healthier for everyone. Cody pondered a bit, then suggested that they make a fruit salad together, and that everyone could choose their favorite fruit to go in it. Anne clapped her hands and laughed. "That's the spirit!" she exclaimed.

continued on page 114

lack the necessary enzymes. There are three kinds of fiber we eat on a regular basis — cellulose, hemicellulose, and pectin. Eating a wide range of fruits, vegetables, legumes, and whole grains will ensure that enough of the various types of fiber is present in the diet.

Fiber is actually a complex carbohydrate. For example, some animals and insects can digest cellulose into its building blocks. Both cows and termites have no problem with it because they have bacteria in their digestive systems secreting enzymes that break down cellulose into glucose. Humans do not have the enzymes (nor the bacteria that make the enzymes) that break down fiber. That is why for us, cellulose is just fiber.

Often the food that contains a lot of fiber also contains a lot of water. It is the fiber that holds the water in the food and causes these foods to occupy more space in the stomach. The other effect of fiber is that it keeps water around it, making the fiber more solid and causing it to occupy more space in the stomach. Liquid without fiber rushes through the stomach very quickly.

Kinds of Fiber

Cellulose
Cellulose is the structural component of plants. It gives a vegetable its familiar shape.

Hemicellulose
Hemicellulose is found in the hulls of different grains like wheat. Wheat bran, for example, is hemicellulose.

Pectin
Pectin is found most often in fruits. It is called a soluble fiber because it dissolves and forms a gel when mixed with water.

Energy Density

The energy density of a food is the amount of energy for a specific weight of food. Remember that 1 gram of fat (9 kcal) has twice the energy as 1 gram of protein (4 kcal) or 1 gram of carbohydrate (4 kcal). This means that fat has more energy density than proteins and carbohydrate.

Energy density can be used to describe the number of calories per gram of whole foods. For example, the energy density of an apple would be the number of kcals for each gram of apple. Many foods are a combination of the three energy-providing macronutrients, so their energy density depends on the amount of fat, carbohydrate, and protein present in each gram of the food. Energy-dense foods have more calories in each gram of the food than low-energy density food. Foods high in fat will be more energy dense because fat has more than twice the energy per gram than does carbohydrate or protein. Water and fiber add no additional energy to the food but they do add more weight and size.

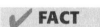 **FACT**

Energy Density Rule
The higher the water and fiber content in food, the lower its energy density. Low-energy density food is more filling and discourages overeating.

Water and Fiber Content
Water content is the reason why fruit and vegetables weigh so much and take up so much space. Water content also has a major effect on the energy density of food. To help you understand this, we will use an example.

Let's consider the energy density of a pure carbohydrate, such as sugar. Its energy density is 4 Calories per gram. Imagine your child eats 1 gram (about ¼ teaspoon) of drink mix crystals (which is mostly pure sugar). One gram of the drink mix crystals gives your child 4 Calories. Now, imagine what would happen if instead of eating them, they were dissolved in a cup of water to make a drink. One cup of water is about 250 ml and weighs around 250 grams. Water is not a macronutrient and has no energy. No matter how much water you use, the only energy in the drink will be from the drink crystals.

But now the energy density has changed. The energy density of the new drink is 4 Calories (from the crystals) in 251 grams of drink (250 grams of water and 1 gram of crystals). Each gram of the drink now has only 0.016 Calories. The crystals eaten alone had 4 Calories per gram. So, the new drink is 250 times less energy dense than the crystals alone.

Apples and Cookies

When the water content of a food is increased, the energy density of the food is decreased. Also, a full cup of water with 1 gram of drink crystals provides the same energy as 1 gram of drink crystals eaten straight. The difference is that your stomach feels fuller after drinking a cup of water with the crystals. The feeling of fullness or satiety doesn't last very long because the fluid quickly rushes through the stomach.

Now let's look at an example of eating food with fiber in addition to water and sugar, for example, an apple. Eating an apple takes a while because each bite is small and has to be chewed before it is swallowed. Because the fiber, combined with water, takes longer to move through the stomach, you will feel a lot fuller and will stay feeling full a lot longer than after eating just sugar or sugar mixed with water alone.

Now, let's imagine eating apples versus cookies. Six small cookies have about 300 calories, whereas three whole apples have 300 calories. You could imagine your child eating six small cookies at one time while sitting in front of the television, with room to eat more. Now imagine him eating the equivalent calories from apples. Eating three apples would make your child feel incredibly full. Eating just one apple would likely make your child feel full but would only give one-third of the calories of a typical portion of cookies. Plus, apples would be providing important vitamins and minerals.

Fiber Removal

Removing fiber from food through processing has an effect on its energy density. Food processing can also change the way foods are digested in the body. This is especially significant in the processing of carbohydrate sources like grain products.

> ✔ **FACT**
>
> **Limiting Overeating**
> Feeling full sooner while eating, and for longer afterward, can help limit overeating. It can also help prevent us from feeling so hungry that we make poor food choices.

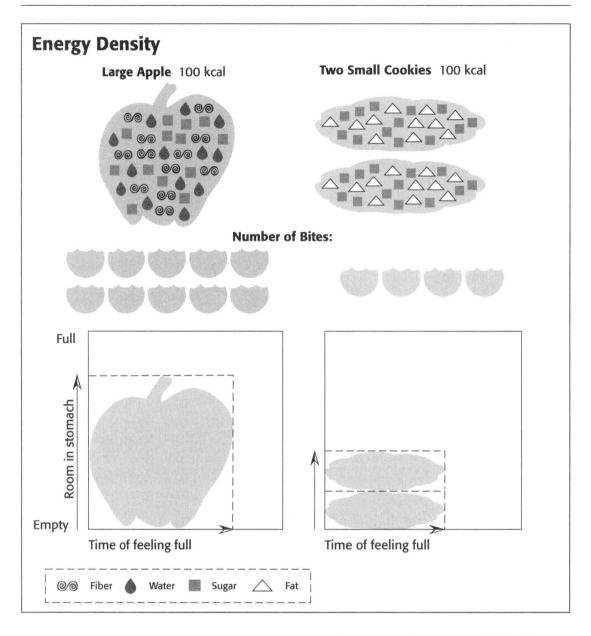

Energy Density

Large Apple 100 kcal   **Two Small Cookies** 100 kcal

Number of Bites:

Full

Room in stomach

Empty

Time of feeling full   Time of feeling full

◎/◎ Fiber   💧 Water   ■ Sugar   △ Fat

Let's compare what happens when your child drinks a can of pop/soda, when your child eats a whole-grain piece of bread, and when your child eats a piece of white bread (made from refined flour).

Soft drinks and fruit drinks are sweetened with glucose and/or fructose, another simple sugar. There is nothing for the body to break down because these carbohydrates are already in their most basic building block form. Because they are a liquid, they can move quickly throughout the digestive system. The sugar is instantly absorbed into the blood stream.

Unlike soft drinks and fruit drinks, the starches in the

Fiber Comparison

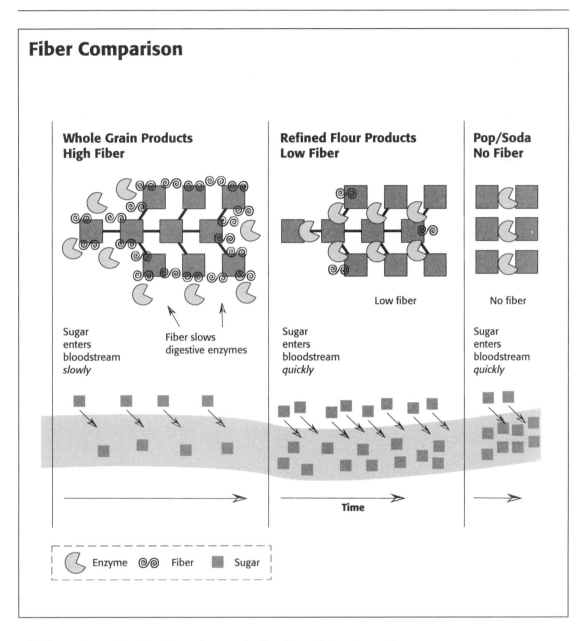

Whole Grain Products High Fiber

Sugar enters bloodstream *slowly*

Fiber slows digestive enzymes

Refined Flour Products Low Fiber

Low fiber

Sugar enters bloodstream *quickly*

Pop/Soda No Fiber

No fiber

Sugar enters bloodstream *quickly*

Time

Enzyme   Fiber   Sugar

whole-grain and white bread must be broken down into glucose before they enter the bloodstream. Whole-grain bread has a lot more fiber than white bread does. Fiber protects the complex carbohydrate from the digestive enzymes, so it takes longer to be broken down into glucose. The more processing of the flour used in any product, the less time it takes for it to be broken down. When whole-grain products are eaten, it takes time for their breakdown into glucose and it takes time for the glucose to enter the bloodstream. Eating refined flour products is similar to eating pure sugar because their breakdown into glucose happens so quickly that sugar can readily enter the bloodstream.

✔ FACT

Overweight and Diabetes

Being overweight is a risk factor for developing diabetes in adolescence. In both children and adults, overweight can make the body less sensitive to the effects of insulin. This means that more insulin is needed to bring blood sugar levels closer to normal after a meal rich in carbohydrates. The decreased sensitivity to insulin and increased demand on the pancreas for insulin can lead to diabetes.

Blood Sugar Regulation

The body attempts to keep the level of glucose in the blood fairly constant at all times. After a meal, the carbohydrates are broken down into their basic building blocks, mostly glucose, and that glucose begins to enter the bloodstream. This causes the glucose levels in the blood to rise. Because the body wants to keep a steady amount of glucose in the blood, an organ in our abdomen called the pancreas releases a hormone called insulin. Insulin allows the body's cells to quickly absorb excess glucose from the blood and return the blood levels back to normal.

Different parts of the body respond differently to blood glucose. Some cells, such as brain cells and nerve cells, can always take as much glucose from the blood as they need. Other cells, such as liver cells, muscle cells, and fat cells, need help to absorb glucose from the blood.

Although digestion of both simple and complex carbohydrates ultimately results in increased glucose in the bloodstream, the rate of entry of glucose into the bloodstream affects the way our body responds. If blood glucose levels rise too quickly, too much insulin can be secreted. If too much insulin is secreted, the blood glucose levels can fall to levels that are too low. One of the responses of the body to low blood glucose levels is the release of adrenaline, a hormone that can cause nervousness and irritability.

The Glycemic Index

Some foods and drinks that have a high amount of simple sugars have what is called a high glycemic index. This relates to how efficiently and quickly they are broken down and absorbed into the bloodstream.

Eating high glycemic index foods, such as candy and soft drinks, are like adding jet fuel to the blood — they are absorbed quickly and efficiently — which results in dramatic

Q: **How can my child keep blood sugar constant and insulin levels low?**

A: When we eat fiber containing foods and whole-grain products, the rise in blood glucose is slower and the insulin release is more appropriate and controlled, ensuring that the blood glucose levels do not fall too low.

responses from the body. Low glycemic index foods, which are higher in fiber (such as most vegetables and whole-grain foods), are like burning wood — the energy release is slower and more constant.

The Healthy Weight Program

With a solid grasp of the basics of energy balance and energy density, you are ready to make informed food choices for your child and for your family as a whole. Choosing food that can restore a healthy body weight for your child is the subject of the next two chapters, which feature a guided tour of the fresh food and processed food sections of your local grocery store. The practical food tips we offer should help you to get a healthy weight for your child.

> ✔ **FACT**
>
> **Low Glycemic Food Benefits**
>
> In some recent studies, where overweight adolescents ate predominantly low glycemic foods, there were improvements in their weight and the complications of overweight.

CASE STUDY Ryan's Family

Owning Up

For the first time Sandra realized her responsibility in this whole situation with Ryan. The Grade 4 bullies were not the only ones to blame. She made Ryan's lunch every morning, and it was her who filled it with goodies. She did this because Ryan loved those treats. He used to tell her how all the kids said he had the best lunches. This always made her feel so good. She was a "cool" mom who made awesome lunches. Sandra never took the time to consider how these foods were contributing to Ryan's weight, and how his weight would affect his self-esteem and health.

Looking at her son now she recognized that he was overweight; it was obvious. So was his father. It was in the genes, right? Or was that just an excuse? How could she have

missed it? Ryan's food choices and increasing overweight were a result of her and Greg not emphasizing or leading a healthy lifestyle. Sandra knew then and there that changes needed to be made. If not, the problem would only get worse.

Sandra looked at her son. "Ryan, just remember that it's what's on the inside that counts the most. You're a great kid from the inside out and people see this first. But I just realized that some of the choices we make as a family are not helping us to lead healthy, strong lives. Your father and I want you and your brother to grow up to be healthy, fit, and active people who are confident and happy. So maybe it's time to make some changes. What do you think?"

continued on page 172

CHAPTER 5

Healthy Weight Food Choices

Part 1: Fresh Whole Foods

The choices you make while shopping are very important in helping your child achieve and maintain a healthy weight. However, choosing good food is challenging, both time-consuming at first and confusing at times given the wide variety of food available in a grocery store.

The weekly trip to the grocery store can often seem like a chore. While trying to make healthy food choices for your family, you are bombarded by advertising for the latest fancy 'snacks' or 'meals' boasting their convenience. The ends of each grocery aisle are capped with various sale-priced goodies. The kids, if you brought them with you, are begging for these cookies, that cereal, and this new drink. If that isn't enough, you are also under time constraints. While you wait in line to check out, once again the snacks available at the counter call out to your kids.

By providing your children with mainly healthy food options, you will be taking a major step toward helping them to achieve and keep a healthy weight. Learning to shop smarter will save you time in the grocery store and help the whole family eat better, too.

So, let's pretend were are 'shopping' at a typical grocery store, moving through the store, food group by food group, section by section, aisle by aisle, focusing on the sources of nutrition. We'll provide a number of food tips along the way to help you make the kind of food choices that lead to a healthy weight for your child.

✔ **FACT**

Good Choices
The choices you make in the grocery store have the greatest impact on your child's nutrition because much of the food your child eats will come from home.

Grocery Store Tour

Fresh Whole Foods

The first part of the tour focuses on the importance of buying whole foods with minimum processing. When you go shopping, this should be your focus, too. When you use these foods to prepare your meals, you are providing your family with the most nutrition. Preparing meals from scratch also gives you control over unnecessary calories from fat and sugar, as well as the size of portions. This allows you to follow the Healthy Energy Rule and the Energy Density Rule we discussed in the previous chapters.

Part 1 of the grocery store tour focuses on the following fresh whole foods:

Section 1: Fruit and Vegetables

Section 2: Legumes, Nuts, and Seeds

Section 3: Grains and Tubers: Breads, Rice, Pasta, and Potatoes

Section 4: Meat, Poultry, Fish, Eggs, and Deli

Section 5: Dairy: Milk, Yogurt, and Cheeses

Processed and Preserved Foods

You may feel that you do not have enough time to prepare all meals and snacks at home. It can be hard as a busy parent to avoid all processed and preserved foods. Following our tour of the fresh, whole food sections of the store, we will tour the processed food sections, learning along the way how to read nutrition labels. This skill can then be used to guide you in making smarter food choices when buying processed and preserved convenience foods.

Part 2 of the grocery store tour focuses on the following processed and preserved foods:

Section 1: Cooking Oils

Section 2: Salad Dressings

Section 3: Condiments, Sauces, Spreads, and Dips

Section 4: Frozen Foods

Section 5: Soups

Section 6: Breakfast Foods and Cereals

Section 7: Baked Goods

Section 8: Chips, Chocolates, and Candies

Section 9: Fruit Juices, Fruit Drinks, and Soda/Pop

In the course of the tour, "Food Tips" for gradually improving nutrition and achieving a healthy weight will be offered. After the tour, a convenient "Shopping Tour Summary" highlights important information that you can carry with you whenever you shop for groceries.

Basics of Shopping for Healthy Weight Foods

Eat More:

- Fruits
- Vegetables
- Whole-grain foods
- High-fiber foods

Eat Less:

- Foods made with refined or white flour
- Processed meats
- Saturated fat by limiting processed foods, high-fat dairy foods (cheeses, creams), and high-fat meat
- Candy, chocolates, cookies, cakes
- High-calorie drinks (pop/soda, fruit drinks, sports drinks)
- Foods high in salt

CASE STUDY Anne's Family

Shopping for Health

Anne and Cody were usually the grocery shoppers in the family, but this time she decided it was time to take everyone. Bill and Mark grumbled, "the baseball game is on!" She would not take "no" for an answer, reminded them of their commitment, and suggested that they walk the five blocks to the supermarket. It was a sunny afternoon, and it was great to be outside. Bill could not remember the last time he had walked through the neighborhood.

In the store, Anne gathered everyone around and gave them each a shopping basket. First Anne asked everyone to go to the produce department and each pick out two vegetables. One vegetable had to be green. Anne picked up lettuce and tomatoes, Cody preferred broccoli and carrots, and Bill chose sweet potatoes and celery.

Mark was clearly having a hard time as he eyed the cabbage. He rarely ate vegetables. He wandered up and down the aisles aimlessly, but Bill went over and offered some encouragement. "Was there something you might like to try that you haven't tried before?" Bill asked. Mark eventually picked up an eggplant and some red peppers. While he missed out on the green vegetable, he had made a choice, although Anne was unsure how the eggplant was going to go over.

Then Anne decided to move everyone on to the fruit section. She felt proud that everyone was working so well together, but knew that there were going to be challenges when they hit the snack food and the breakfast cereal sections. She wondered if maybe she should have taught them how to read nutritional labels before she brought them on this first trip.

continued on page 143

Fruit and Vegetables

The first thing you notice in the fresh fruit and vegetable section of the grocery store is the wide range of color. The color actually comes from the range of vitamins and minerals in fruit and vegetables. The darker green, bright red, and orange foods you see in this section are packed full of vitamins and minerals.

Most fruits and vegetables are low in fat and calories. They are a natural source of vitamins, minerals, antioxidants, and fiber that are all beneficial to our health. In addition, they can help prevent us from overeating because they have low energy density and help keep us feeling full for longer. For all of these reasons we should aim to eat lots of fruit and vegetables.

Much is known about the improvement in health and decrease in disease that comes from eating fruit and vegetables regularly and in sufficient amounts. Despite this, they are very often lacking or missing in the diet of many children and adults. Eating a wide variety of foods from this section is one of the most important steps your whole family can take toward improving health. Fruit and vegetables provide us with the micronutrients needed to support every single process that occurs in the body. Without them, it is more difficult to achieve a healthy weight.

Q: **What is a healthy amount of vitamins and minerals?**

A: A diet of fresh, natural food, such as fruit, vegetables, legumes, whole grains and meat products, will usually provide healthy people with all of the vitamins and minerals needed. Processing tends to destroy vitamins and many processed foods need to be 'fortified' with man-made vitamins.

Antioxidant Source

Fresh fruit and vegetables are also a source of antioxidants, micronutrients that help our body get rid of harmful free radicals. Free radicals are a natural product of the chemical reactions that happen in our body. Without antioxidants, the free radicals can actually damage our blood vessels, making them more prone to atherosclerosis. Atherosclerosis is the hardening of the walls of blood vessels caused by the accumulation of fat in the artery wall. The fat deposits can become large and start narrowing arteries, which can ultimately result in a heart attack or stroke. Free radicals also increase the risk of cancers.

Antioxidants protect the cells of our body by eliminating free radicals. They are often called free radical scavengers. The most commonly mentioned antioxidants are vitamin C, vitamin E, beta-carotene (carotenoids), selenium, and polyphenols.

Q: **How much antioxidant micronutrients does my child need?**

A: Guidelines have not been set for the amount and type of antioxidants that are optimal for health. Recently, a major study was undertaken to determine which of 100 commonly eaten foods had the highest levels of antioxidant effects. The findings of that study strongly suggest that it is very important that we include a wide variety of fruit, vegetables, beans, nuts, and even spices in our diet.

Best Sources of Antioxidants

- Fresh fruit: Blueberries, cranberries, blackberries, raspberries, and strawberries have very high levels of antioxidants. High levels are also found in red delicious apples, Granny Smith apples, plums, avocados, and cherries.
- Dried fruit: Prunes have very high levels of antioxidants. Dates, figs, and raisins all have high levels as well.
- Fresh vegetables: Artichoke has the highest levels of antioxidants. Dark, leafy vegetables, such as spinach and lettuces (except iceberg lettuce), all have high levels as well. Raw asparagus, cabbages, and eggplant were also good sources.
- Spices: Cloves, cinnamon, oregano leaf, and turmeric have high levels of antioxidants.

FACT

Chocolate Bonus

Baking chocolate has 10 times higher levels of antioxidants than milk chocolate. The higher the amount of cocoa in the chocolate, the higher the level of antioxidants.

Fiber

You'll notice that as you add items to your cart in the fruit and vegetable section, your cart fills up quickly. Fruit and vegetables take up a lot of room because they have a high water and fiber content. They have low energy density, as we discussed in previous chapters, which is important for filling us up and reaching satiety.

Another important effect of fiber is maintenance of bowel regularity. Recently, studies have found other health benefits as well. Regular consumption of fiber has been shown to be beneficial for some of the medical problems that can be caused by overweight. There is good evidence that dietary fiber helps reduce total cholesterol and LDL cholesterol, which is good news for our cardiovascular system. Higher fiber intake has also been associated with lower blood pressure. There is also strong evidence that fiber protects against type 2 diabetes, another complication of overweight. Fiber causes food to stay in the stomach longer, making us feel full longer. It also decreases the energy density of food. Because of these effects, eating foods high in fiber may be helpful for reducing overeating and preventing unwanted weight gain.

Q: How much fiber does my child need?

A: The daily amount of fiber recommended for children is their AGE + 5 grams. By eating enough fruit, vegetables, legumes, nuts, and whole-grain foods, your child will be getting all the fiber they need. Figs, prunes, and raspberries have the highest fiber content among fresh fruits. Spinach, kale, broccoli, and carrots are high in fiber.

Dried and Canned Fruit

When fresh fruit and vegetable varieties are out of season or not in stock at the grocery stores, dried fruit and canned fruits and vegetables are alternative sources of key micronutrients. They need to be eaten with caution, however, because they are often energy dense (in the case of dried fruit) and packed in sugar or salt solutions.

Dried Fruit

Dried fruit is a convenient and healthy snack but its energy density should be considered here. Most of the water has been removed from these foods, which accounts for their small size and weight, while the carbohydrate remains in the fruit. That means that there are many more calories in a much smaller package and it makes it easier to eat a lot more. To help imagine this, compare eating fresh apricots to dried apricots. It probably isn't hard to imagine eating 5 to 10 dried apricots but eating that many fresh apricots would be very difficult.

Canned Fruit and Vegetables

When purchasing canned fruit, be mindful that it does not have quite the same nutritional value as fresh fruit because some nutrients are destroyed in the processing. Obviously, it is not as tasty either but it is sometimes more economical when fruit is out of season. Likewise, the processing of canned vegetables can sometimes damage some of the nutrition components, so fresh produce is preferred when available and economical.

Portions

The goal for both children and adults should be to have 2 to 3 servings of fruit and at least 3 to 5 servings of vegetables per day. Having more than 5 servings of vegetables is just great.

Even though fruits and vegetables have different nutrient content, the number of different serving sizes is kept to a minimum to make it easy to remember. By eating a variety of fruit and vegetables, you will ensure that an adequate amount of all the nutrients are being eaten.

Variety is essential. By changing the fruit and vegetables eaten day to day or week to week, you help ensure that your child is receiving all the important nutrients they need for good health.

 FACT

Dried Fruit Caution

Dried fruit, such as raisins, can stick to teeth, increasing the risk for cavities. Be sure to brush teeth after eating these foods or chew sugarless gum.

Q: **How much is one serving of fruit and vegetables?**

A: A serving of fruit is considered to be one medium-sized fruit, such as an apple, banana, orange, or pear. One serving of chopped, cooked, or canned fruit is about ½ cup.

A serving of vegetables is considered to be 1 cup of leafy vegetables or about ½ cup of other vegetables, raw or cooked; for example, 1 cup of lettuce or about 8 baby carrots.

Food Tips

- When choosing canned fruit and vegetables, be sure that no extra sugar has been added. Try to avoid cans with labels that say "in syrup." Look instead for cans that are labeled "in its own juice" or "No added sugar."

- When choosing canned vegetables, try to avoid those with too much salt used as a preservative. When possible, strain and wash canned vegetables well to remove excess salt.

- Always keep plenty of ready to eat fruits and vegetables (fresh, frozen, and canned) in the kitchen and in sight.

- Add fresh chopped fruit to cereal, yogurt, pancakes, and muffins.

- Fresh chopped carrots, celery, broccoli, cauliflower, and peppers make great healthy snacks.

- Add fresh greens, carrots, celery, parsley, tomatoes, and/or beans to store-bought or homemade soups.

- Keep dried fruit, such as apricots, figs, dates, and raisins, available as a quick snack.

- Snack on raw vegetables instead of chips, crackers, or chocolate bars.

Legumes, Nuts, and Seeds

Legumes (beans, peas, lentils, soybeans, peanuts), nuts, and seeds are all an excellent source of protein, healthy fats, vitamins, minerals, antioxidants, and phytochemicals. You can often find them in a natural and unprocessed form. Seeds and especially nuts are a great source of healthy mono- and polyunsaturated fats and should be part of a balanced diet. However, because nuts and seeds have a high healthy fat content, they should be eaten in moderation to avoid excessive calories.

Good Protein Source

Legumes, nuts, and seeds are so high in protein that they are referred to as meat alternatives. However, they are not sources of complete proteins because they are low in or are missing some of the amino acid building blocks. If your diet did not include any animal protein sources, it would be necessary to eat legumes, nuts, and seeds in combination with whole-grain foods. Certain whole-grain foods contain the amino acids that are missing from legumes, nuts, and seeds.

Healthy Fats

We can't stress enough that fats are an essential part of the diet. Low-fat foods often replace the fat with extra carbohydrates and are not the solution to the increasing level of overweight in North America. It may be an unrealistic ideal, but if we consumed a diet rich in fruit, vegetables, legumes, nuts, seeds, and whole grains, with moderate amounts of fish, poultry, and lean meat, we would be much less concerned about the amount of fat in our diet.

The average North American does not eat in this way, instead consuming larger and larger amounts of processed and packaged food. The amount of saturated and trans fats in many of these foods has become excessive. Add to this the increase in our carbohydrate consumption over the past decades, and it becomes easy to eat more calories than our body uses up in a day. Although unsaturated and saturated fat have equally high energy density, the fact that unsaturated fats are beneficial for our heart makes them a preferable choice. When we are in energy balance, eating larger amounts of unsaturated fats does not result in excessive weight gain when saturated fats are kept at a reasonable level.

Q: **What is a healthy amount of fat in our diet?**

A: Nutritionists, the American Heart Association, and the Heart and Stroke Foundation of Canada all recommend a diet with less than 30% of calories from fat. They also recommend that no more than 10% of the calories come from saturated fat. Because almost all the saturated fat we eat comes from animals or processed foods, we will discuss the reasonable amounts of these fats when we come to the appropriate sections, where we show how to keep track of the amount of saturated fat in your child's diet.

Saturated versus Unsaturated Fat

Not all fat is bad, though from news reports and fat-free fad diets you might conclude that all fat is bad for the body. It is true that excess saturated fat (the kind found in high-fat meat and whole-fat dairy products) has been shown to increase the risk of heart disease. It is also true that the man-made saturated fats and trans fats found in some margarines and many processed foods are even more harmful. Saturated fats should be limited in the diet.

However, some unsaturated fats are actually good for our body and can even protect us from heart disease. The fat we eat in our diet comes from both plant and animal products. Almost all the fats that come from plant products are unsaturated, either monounsaturated or polyunsaturated. Nuts and seeds are especially high in monounsaturated or polyunsaturated fats.

Two specific types of polyunsaturated fat are the omega-6 and omega-3 fatty acids. They are essential fatty acids (our body can't produce them). They have both been associated with a decrease in heart disease. Omega-3 type fats are very important in the development of the brain.

Q: **What kinds of foods are high in monounsaturated and polyunsaturated fats?**

A: The goal should be to have the unsaturated fats as the largest source of fat in your child's diet.

- Monounsaturated fat sources: Walnuts, almonds, sesame seeds, olive oil, canola oil, avocados.
- Polyunsaturated omega-3 fatty acids: Walnuts, pecans and pine nuts, flaxseed, soybean oils, fattier fish (mackerel, herring, trout, salmon, swordfish, cod, and bluefish).
- Polyunsaturated omega-6 fatty acids: Legumes, nuts, seeds, soybean, as well as sesame, sunflower, safflower, and corn oils. Processing of vegetable oils that contain omega-6 fatty acids gives them a longer shelf life, but the processing often damages them.

Fiber and Antioxidants

In addition to being an excellent source of protein and fat, legumes, nuts, and seeds are also an excellent source of fiber and antioxidants. Among the legumes, beans have high antioxidant levels, including pinto beans, black beans, navy beans, red kidney beans, and small red beans. Among the nuts, pecans have the highest levels of antioxidant levels, though walnuts, hazelnuts, and pistachios also have high levels.

Q: **What kind of peanut butter is best?**

A: Peanut butter is an excellent source of protein and can be a great source of healthy fat. It is also a great food because children often like the taste. When selecting peanut butter, choose natural peanut butter. Processed peanut butter can include extra sugar and salt, as well as hydrogenated oils and possibly trans fats. Other seeds and nuts are excellent choices, but they can loose their nutritive value when processed. The roasting process can damage important nutrients and often salt and extra oils are added.

Portions

The goal for both children and adults should be to eat some of these foods on a daily basis. In fact, it is recommended that whole meals be based around meat alternatives, such as legumes two or more days of the week. By eating these foods, along with whole-grain foods, it is very easy to meet daily protein needs.

Q: **How much is one serving of legumes, nuts, and seeds?**

A: One serving of beans is about ½ cup of raw beans or cooked dry beans.

One serving of nuts or seeds is about ¼ cup. The portion size of these foods is smaller because they have a high protein and healthy fat content and because they have high energy density.

The serving sizes for legumes, nuts, and seeds are based on the same protein and mineral content as 1 oz (30 g) of meat and provides about 7 to 10 grams of protein.

Food Tips

- Try to buy seeds and nuts that are raw and unprocessed without added salt or oils. They are likely more expensive but the nutritive value outweighs the additional cost.

- Always keep raw seeds and nuts in the kitchen for a quick nutritious snack. Remember that only a small portion is needed.

- Substitute legumes for meat two to three times a week in chili and soups.

- Use walnuts, sesame seeds, and other nuts and seeds in moderation for a salad topping instead of croutons or bacon.

Grains and Tubers

Grain and tuber foods include wheat, oats, rice, and potatoes, as well as the flours and products produced from these flours, such as breads and pastas. These grains and tubers all have carbohydrate as their main macronutrient. They are starches, complex carbohydrates or chains of simple sugars linked together. When we eat foods rich in complex carbohydrates, our digestive system must break them down into their component building blocks, the sugars, before they can be absorbed into our bloodstream.

It may surprise you to learn that studies of North American food consumption over the past 50 years show that we are consuming more and more carbohydrates, but the total amount of fat and protein we eat has remained about the same. Many North Americans consume too much carbohydrate, specifically processed and refined carbohydrates.

Remember the Positive Energy Rule: all extra calories, even when they come from carbohydrates, get converted to body fat.

White Grain Rule

Remember from our visit to the fruit and vegetable section that the lush color of these foods tells us that they are packed with important vitamins, minerals, and phytochemicals. When those colors are missing from our processed foods, so are the natural nutrients. Try to think of fresh, whole foods that are white. There are few naturally white, whole foods.

Many processed grains are white, the products of an agricultural revolution. While people have eaten grain products for centuries and centuries, the amount of processing of the grains has increased so significantly in the past 50 years that eating many of these grain products is, in fact, exactly like eating pure sugar. The quick rise in blood sugar after eating highly processed grain products is not healthy for our body.

Processing of grains can strip away the fiber and the nutrients they contain. In addition, processing makes the starch more readily available to your digestive system. When we eat grain products that are less processed, such as whole wheat or whole-grain products, the starches are better protected by their fiber from the enzymes in our stomach. This makes the breakdown of the starches a slower process.

 FACT

Paying Attention

If we are concerned about our children's health, we must pay more attention to the quality of the grain products we are feeding them. Aim to serve whole grains, not 'white' grains. Use the White Grain Rule to improve nutrition by slowly replacing white processed flour, rice, and potato with other less processed varieties. The natural nutrients that are stripped away in the processing of the various grain products are definitely important for health.

FACT

Insulin Boost
Whole-grain food intake has been found to increase the effects of insulin in middle-aged adults.

 FACT

Whole or Not
When bread products have packaging that says "whole grain," this does not necessarily mean that they are made from whole grain flour. Looking on the ingredient list is the only way to know for sure. Terms like "enriched flour," "enriched wheat flour," and "unbleached wheat flour" all mean that refined white flour is being used. Look for "Whole" in the first few ingredients of the ingredients list.

Baked goods, such as white breads, pastries, crackers, and cookies, are most often made with flour from highly processed wheat. The wheat is often so highly processed that when we eat these products, the white flour is instantly converted to glucose. This means that eating them is just like drinking sugar-sweetened drinks or eating candy.

Wheat Products
The White Grain Rule applies to processed wheat. Wheat is a member of the grass family that has been used as a food source for thousands of years. Whole civilizations have depended on wheat for their livelihood. Whole wheat kernels (wheat berries) are ground into flour for use in bread, tortillas, pasta, noodles, cakes, breakfast cereals, cookies, and crackers. To store large quantities of flour for long periods of time, grain processing removes part of the kernel that would make the flour spoil. Processing removes the nutrient-rich outer bran and germ layers, as well as the oils of the wheat berry.

These are the layers that contain most of the important fats, vitamins (such as vitamin E) and minerals. A bleaching process is often used to treat proteins and other nutrients in some of the flour to extend further the flour's shelf life. The processed flour is commonly 'enriched' as a last step by adding back same types of nutrients that were removed in processing, but in smaller amounts and possible deficient in phytochemicals.

Rice Products
The White Grain Rule applies to rice. Processing of rice involves the removal of the nutrient rich portion of the rice grain and makes the rice more like pure sugar. The only difference between white rice and brown is processing. Rice with the hulls removed but the bran left on is brown rice. White rice is further processed by polishing and 'enriching' it.

The nutritional value of rice is concentrated in the outer layers (bran) of the granule that are removed in the polishing step converting brown rice to white rice. These outer layers are rich in B-vitamins, vitamin E, minerals, fiber, and fats. Enrichment of white rice involves spraying vitamins and minerals onto the rice. A significant amount of protein, fiber, fats, and phytochemicals removed during processing may not be replaced.

> ✔ **FACT • Low-Carb Diets**
>
> Recently, low-carb diets have become very popular. These diets often involve cutting out a majority of the grain products. However, there are no medical studies showing long-term safety of a diet that is low in carbohydrates but high in protein and, often, saturated fat. We don't promote severe restrictions of carbohydrates in food. It is the quality of the carbohydrate sources that is more important.

Potatoes

The White Grain Rule applies to potatoes. When they are processed, they lose their nutrients and become more like pure sugar.

Potatoes are part of the tuber family of food. They have only become a main staple for North Americans in the last hundred or so years. The reason we are mentioning them here is because they share one important feature with the grains. Regular potatoes have some vitamins and minerals but they are loaded with starch. This means that they can easily contribute a large number of calories and make us feel too full to eat other nutrient-rich foods. When they are fried, they soak up oils and become even more energy dense.

Portions

The recommendations for the number of servings of the carbohydrate foods are 5 to 11 servings per day. Ideally, all carbohydrates should be coming from whole-grain sources.

Q: **How much is one healthy serving of commonly eaten carbohydrate foods?**

A: Learning about how much food is considered a serving is one way to ensure that you are not overconsuming carbohydrates. The serving sizes for the grain products were chosen so that they would be approximately equivalent to the nutrient content and calories of one thin slice of bread (between 50 and 100 calories).

- 1 thin slice of bread
- 3 inch bread roll
- ½ regular size bagel
- ½ regular pita bread
- ½ regular muffin
- 1 cup of breakfast cereal
- ¾ cup of oatmeal
- ½ cup of cooked rice
- ½ cup of mashed potatoes
- ½ cup of cooked pasta

Food Tips

- Spend time looking for products made from whole grains, such as whole grain breads, rolls, and bagels, as well as whole-grain pizza crusts, tortillas, wraps, and pitas. Also experiment with new and healthier grains made from whole wheat, for example, bulgur, quinoa, buckwheat, and millet.

- Try less processed rice varieties, such as brown long-grain, whole grain, and wild rice blends. Brown rice takes a little longer to cook and has a nutty flavor.

- Look for pasta made from less processed flours, such as whole wheat, quinoa, spelt, buckwheat, semolina, and brown rice flour.

- Try using a measuring cup to serve pasta or rice so that the number of servings is easily known.

Meat, Poultry, Fish, Eggs, and Deli

Meat, poultry, fish, and eggs are all excellent sources of complete protein. That means that they provide all the amino acid building blocks our body needs to make new proteins. These foods are also an excellent source of iron, which is essential for delivering oxygen throughout our body. When buying these products, our main concern is the amount of saturated fat they contain. Often deli meat is very high in saturated fats, not to mention salt, preservatives, and nitrates, which are all considered unhealthy. The foods mentioned in this section are all sources of large amounts of protein. Many other foods have small amounts of protein that add up quite a bit throughout the day. These foods include whole-grain products and dairy products.

Good Sources of Iron

Iron is used in our red blood cells to allow them to pick up oxygen from the air we breathe and deliver it throughout our body. Iron is present in foods in two different forms, heme iron and non-heme iron. The heme iron form is found in animal meats and fish. It is the easiest for the body to use. The non-heme iron is found in plant products. It is more difficult for our body to absorb. Iron is also added to many cereals and other processed foods.

Even though vegetables, legumes, and whole grains may have high iron content, we cannot necessarily absorb all of it, but when we eat these foods along with animal meats, we improve the absorption of the non-heme iron. Another way to increase the amount of non-heme iron we absorb is by adding foods containing vitamin C (ascorbic acid) to the meal, such as citrus fruits (grapefruit, oranges, lemons, limes), tomatoes, strawberries, potatoes, broccoli, cauliflower, and spinach.

Common Sources of Iron		
Heme Iron Sources	**Amount**	**Iron Content (mg)**
Lean ground beef	125 g	3.4
Beef (bottom round)	125 g	3.3
Shrimp	90 g	2.3
Tuna fish (canned in water)	125 g	1.9
Poultry (without skin)	125 g	1.8
Non-Heme Iron Sources		
Cream of Wheat cereal (cooked with water)	1 cup	10.2
Instant oatmeal	1 packet	3.8
Whole-grain and fortified cereals, breads, drinks	Varies	See nutrient label
Lentils (boiled)	1 cup	6.6
Spinach (boiled, drained)	1 cup	6.4
Kidney beans (boiled)	1 cup	5.2
Barley	1 cup	5.0
Chickpeas (boiled)	1 cup	4.7
Navy beans (boiled)	1 cup	4.5
Soybeans (boiled)	1 cup	4.5
Lima beans (boiled)	1 cup	4.5
Pumpkin seeds (roasted)	1 oz	4.2
Dark, leafy greens	1 cup	Varies

Adapted from: Dietary Guidelines for Americans, 2005. USDA and U.S. Department of Agriculture, Agricultural Research Service. 2004. USDA Nutrient Database for Standard References, Release 17. Nutrient Data Laboratory. www.nal.usda.gov/fnic/foodcomp

Q: **How much iron does my child need?**

A: Insufficient iron in the diet can lead to a condition called iron-deficiency anemia, which simply means that there is a lack of iron in the blood. Even mild deficiencies can result in fatigue, irritability, dizziness, weakness, and even impaired learning.

Recommended amount of total daily iron:

Children aged 1-3:	7 mg/d
Children aged 4-8:	10 mg/d
Youth aged 9-13:	8 mg/d
Males aged 14-18:	11 mg/d
Females aged 14-18:	15 mg/d

The daily recommendations for iron are guidelines only. It is quite possible that less than the recommended amount will be consumed on a few days of the week and more than the recommended amount will be consumed on other days. This is fine because the body is very good at leveling out these differences.

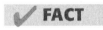

✔ FACT

Reduce Saturated Fats

The body can make its own saturated fat and we don't need to make a point of eating enough. To reduce the risks of too much saturated fat, aim to eat foods with a minimum amount.

Saturated Fat

Almost all saturated fat in the foods we eat comes from animal and man-made sources. The animal source of saturated fat is body fat, the type of fat that animals and people use to store excess energy. In animals, most of the saturated fat lies over muscle and just below the skin, just like human body fat. In addition, fat is deposited inside animal muscle tissue. The muscle tissue of an animal is what we call meat.

Man-made saturated fats are created by processing unsaturated vegetable fats into saturated fat, making them solid at room temperature. For example, vegetable shortening is vegetable oil that has been processed into a solid form.

Cholesterol Health Risks

We should limit the amount of saturated fat we eat because many studies have shown that saturated fats contribute to heart disease. Being overweight and eating a diet high in saturated fat can further increase the chances of having a heart attack or stroke. One of the reasons that a diet high in saturated fat may increase the likelihood of heart disease is that it can cause our blood cholesterol levels to rise.

> ### ✔ FACT • Cholesterol Free
>
> High cholesterol is a risk factor for developing heart disease. Overweight people often have unhealthy levels of cholesterol in the blood. Plant products (including plant fats) don't have any cholesterol.

Cholesterol is a part of the cell wall of every single cell in our body and used by the body to make hormones. Cholesterol comes in two major forms: the HDL type (also called the 'good' or 'Healthy' cholesterol), which we want to be Higher, and the LDL type (also called the 'bad' cholesterol), which we want to be Lower.

LDL cholesterol has a tendency to become deposited in the walls of our blood vessels. This happens even in young children. The HDL cholesterol has the ability to clean up LDL cholesterol from the blood vessel walls. When HDL levels are low, they can't clean up enough cholesterol. When LDL levels are high, too much cholesterol is deposited and can eventually lead to a complete block of the blood vessel. When a blood vessel to the heart is blocked, you can have a heart attack. When a blood vessel to the brain is blocked, you can have a stroke.

The body gets cholesterol in two ways. Our liver can make all the cholesterol we need, but we also get cholesterol from the animal products that we eat, including meat, whole milk (not low-fat dairy products), and egg yolks.

Q: How do I reduce saturated fat in my child's diet?

A: Because saturated fat can often be seen, we can avoid eating it, though once meat or poultry is heated, some of the saturated fat can become liquid and will be difficult to avoid unless it is drained away. To avoid this problem, choose cuts of meat with less visible fat and trim away the white fat you see around meat and poultry before cooking. When using poultry, removing the skin before cooking will significantly lower the amount of saturated fat in the meal. If you are making stews and soups using animal products or even when they are bought in a store or restaurant bought, cooling them in the fridge will solidify the saturated fat and allow you to remove it from the top before re-heating it.

Q: **How do we get too much LDL cholesterol in our blood?**

A: **Genes:** Genes play a major role in determining how much cholesterol is in the blood. Some people get genes from their parents (who likely have high cholesterol) that can result in poor clearance of LDL from the blood or not enough HDL production. Children with high cholesterol have a higher chance of developing heart disease as they grow older.

Food: Recent research shows that the amount of cholesterol in the food we eat has less effect on our blood cholesterol than once thought. Instead, the amount of saturated, trans fats, and unsaturated fat eaten are more important in affecting cholesterol levels. High amounts of saturated and trans fats in the diet (and being overweight) often lead to high LDL cholesterol. However, eating more unsaturated fat and less saturated fat can actually lead to lower LDL cholesterol and even increase HDL cholesterol. For heart health, all people should limit the amount of saturated and trans fats in the diet and eat mostly unsaturated fats.

White Fat Rule

The meat and poultry section is another area in the grocery store where we want to avoid "white." The white you see in any of the meat or poultry is mostly saturated fat. You can see it all around the edges of some meat and poultry. Also notice that in meat you can often see white spots or lines within the meat itself. This is also saturated fat. There is a small amount of saturated fat on the inside of poultry, which is difficult to see.

In ground meat or deli meats, a lot of saturated fat may be seen or it may be hidden. The white spots you see in ground beef or in salami slices is saturated fat. Sometimes meat or poultry, along with its saturated fat, are ground so fine that you can't tell the meat from the fat. This is especially true with poultry because it is precooked and white, making it even more difficult to notice fat. The skin of poultry is very high in saturated fat, although, again, it may be difficult for you to see it.

✔ **FACT**

Egg a Day
According to the American Heart Association, one egg yolk every single day is healthy if other foods high in saturated fats and cholesterol are kept to a minimum.

Q: **What kinds of animal products are low in saturated fats?**

A: **Whole Meat:** Fresh meat products with more than 10% fat can be considered high in fat. The fat in these products is mostly saturated. Eating high-fat meat can easily lead to excessive calorie intake and too much saturated fat. Aim to eat lean fresh meat (less than 5% fat).

Deli Meat: Deli meats are processed meats that are often very high in saturated fat, as well as salt, nitrates, and other ingredients used to preserve the meat and give it flavor. It is always better to use whole meats that are sliced thin for sandwiches. This way, you know what is going into the slices and unnecessary ingredients are avoided. When giving up deli is not an option, lower fat meats should be chosen (5% or less fat).

Poultry: Poultry also has saturated fat but in much smaller amounts than meat if the skin is removed.

Fish: Saturated fat is solid at room temperature. Fish swim in temperatures much colder than room temperature, so their fat must be unsaturated. Fish are an excellent source of unsaturated fat. They are also a great source of the omega-3 fats essential for good health. Some examples of fish with higher levels of the good omega-3 fat include salmon, trout, herring, mackerel, sardines, and albacore tuna (packed in water).

Eggs: All the fuss about cholesterol over the years has made people more concerned about eggs. Egg yokes do contain saturated fat and cholesterol, so eating them in large numbers may not be healthy. However, eggs are inexpensive, low in calories, and a good source of complete protein. They are rich in important nutrients, such as vitamin A, vitamin B-12, vitamin D, vitamin K, folate, riboflavin, and selenium. In fact, the fat in eggs helps our bodies absorb more of the nutrients present. The fat, cholesterol, and vitamins are located specifically in the yolk of eggs, whereas the whites have all the protein. Using egg whites in combination with whole eggs is an easy way to add quality protein to the diet. Substituting two egg whites for each whole egg in recipes is also an excellent idea.

Saturated Fat Content of Common Meats, Poultry, and Seafood

	Amount (g)	Total Fat (g)	Saturated Fat (g)
Ground Meat			
Regular ground beef (25% fat)	100	25.0	9.5
Lean ground beef (10% fat)	100	10.0	4.1
Extra lean ground beef (5% fat)	100	5.0	2.2
Ground turkey	100	8.3	2.3
Deli Meat			
Beef thin-sliced	30	1.1	0.5
Beef bologna	30	7.9	3.1
Pork bologna	30	5.6	1.9
Pepperoni	30	11.3	4.5
Ham	30	2.4	0.8
Beef			
Short loin, porterhouse steak	100	17.3	6.8
Top sirloin	100	12.7	5.1
Beef chuck pot roast	100	18.0	7.3
Pork			
Bacon (medium sliced)	100	45.0	15.0
Wiener (pork, turkey)	45	29.9	9.5
Pork loin chop (boneless)	100	6.3	2.8
Poultry			
Chicken breast (skinless, boneless)	100	1.2	0.3
Chicken breast (with skin)	100	9.3	2.7
Turkey breast (with skin)	100	7.0	1.9
Turkey (light meat with skin)	100	7.4	2.0
Turkey (light meat without skin)	100	1.6	0.5
Turkey (dark meat with skin)	100	8.8	2.6
Seafood			
Light tuna fish (canned in water)	100	0.8	0.2
Pink salmon (canned)	100	6.1	1.5
Wild Atlantic salmon	100	6.3	1.0

	Amount (g)	Total Fat (g)	Saturated Fat (g)
Seafood (cont.)			
Atlantic cod	100	0.7	0.1
Snapper	100	1.3	0.3
Mackerel	100	13.9	3.3
Halibut	100	2.3	0.3
Shrimp	100	1.7	0.3

Adapted from: Dietary Guidelines for Americans, 2005. USDA and U.S. Department of Agriculture, Agricultural Research Service. 2004. USDA Nutrient Database for Standard References, Release 17. Nutrient Data Laboratory. www.nal.usda.gov/fnic/foodcomp

High/Low Saturated Fats

The following is a list of the types of animal products that are high in saturated fat and low in saturated fat, respectively.

Products high in fat:

Beef: High-fat hamburger, short ribs, brisket, corned beef, ground sirloin, ground chuck

Veal: Breast, stew meat, flank

Pork: Sausage, bacon, spareribs

Poultry: Any with skin

Deli: Loaf lunch meats, beef bologna, pepperoni, salami, beef and pork link sausage, beef and pork frankfurter, any sausage

Products lower in fat:

Beef: Extra-lean ground meat, sirloin and round cuts (5% or less fat)

Poultry: Skinless turkey and chicken breast

Pork: lean

Veal: lean

Deli: Meat that lists 5% or less fat

Portions

An average 10-year-old child who eats a bowl of cereal with milk at breakfast, a peanut butter sandwich for lunch, and a very small amount of chicken at dinner would have all the protein needed for the day.

The recommendations for meat, poultry, fish, eggs and/or meat alternatives (such as legumes, nuts, and seeds) are 2 to 3 servings per day. Children's protein needs increase as they grow into adults. One serving for a younger child can be 50 grams of lean meat, poultry, or fish, or one egg. One serving for an older child or teenager can be 100 grams of lean meat, poultry, or fish, or two eggs.

Q: **How much is one serving of meat, poultry, fish, or eggs?**

A: **Meat, Poultry, and Fish:** One serving is around 2 to 3 ounces (around 50 to 100 grams), about the size of a deck of cards. The serving size for a younger child will be at the lower end of this range and for an older child, it will be up at the higher end of the range.

Eggs: One serving of eggs is between 1 and 2 eggs. For a younger child, one egg would count as a serving, for a teenager, 2 eggs would count as one serving.

Meat Alternatives: 2 tablespoons of peanut butter is considered one serving
½ to 1 cup of legumes is considered one serving
⅓ cup of tofu is considered one serving

The serving sizes for alternatives were set to be equivalent to the amount of protein in 1 ounce (30 g) of meat, poultry, or fish. One serving of alternatives provides about 7 to 10 grams of protein.

Food Tips

- Lean cuts of meat are those with the words "loin" or "round" in the name. Examples include sirloin, tenderloin, top round, and ground round.

- When buying meat, choose "lean" or "extra lean" cuts more often. "Lean" indicates that the meat has less than 10 grams of fat (<10%), less than 4.5 grams of which is saturated, and less than 95 milligrams of cholesterol per 100g serving. "Extra lean" indicates that the meat has less than 5 grams of fat (<5%), less than 2 grams of which is saturated, and less than 95 milligrams of cholesterol per serving.

- When using poultry, removing the skin before cooking will significantly lower the amount of saturated fat in the meal.

- Because saturated fat can often be seen in meat and poultry products, we can avoid eating it, though once meat or poultry is heated, some of the saturated fat can become liquid and will be difficult to avoid unless it is drained away. To avoid this problem, choose cuts of meat with less visible fat and trim away the white fat you see around meat and poultry before cooking.

- Prepare low-fat meatless meals more than twice a week. Ensure adequate protein by using legumes, nuts, seeds, eggs, and low-fat cheese.

- Prepare mixed dishes with vegetables, beans, rice (preferably brown), or whole-wheat pasta mixed with small amounts of extra-lean meat. Some examples include stir-fries, chili, spaghetti sauce, soups, and casseroles.

Dairy: Milk, Yogurt, and Cheeses

Most of us grew up with constant reminders about the importance of calcium to build strong teeth and bones. Dairy products are in fact an excellent source of both calcium and protein. In addition, milk often has vitamin D added, which is especially important in most of North America, where people get less sun exposure, especially in the winter. Calcium and vitamin D are essential for developing strong bones and teeth in growing children.

> **✔ FACT**
>
> **Calcium Content**
> Each cup of milk (250 ml) provides one-quarter to one-third of the daily recommended calcium intake. Other dairy products are also excellent sources of calcium.

However, dairy products can also be a source of saturated fats. Recently, the evidence that saturated fat is harmful to the cardiovascular system has raised public awareness. The dairy industry has responded by introducing a wide range of low-fat dairy products. Nutritionists in North America now promote these lower-fat options to the public.

There are two main reasons that North Americans eat dairy products. Many people enjoy the taste, especially the taste of the higher-fat dairy products. Often, foods with more fat appeal more to us. Because of the high amount of saturated fat and calories in some of these foods, we have to pay attention to the size of our portions so that we do not over-consume. We also eat dairy products because we want to ensure that we are getting enough calcium for strong bones and teeth. The ideal amount of calcium we need in our diet has never been determined and research is continuing in this area. Nonetheless, age and gender specific recommendations have been made for calcium. For now, the healthiest option is to eat a wide variety of calcium-containing foods (dairy or non-dairy) each day.

Non-Dairy Sources of Calcium

Calcium is available from a variety of natural non-dairy sources and in foods that have been supplemented with additional calcium. Some commonly eaten foods that are high in calcium include legumes (such as black beans, white beans, soybeans, navy beans, chickpeas), vegetables (such as broccoli, squash, kale, spinach, Swiss chard) and tofu. Many beverages are also fortified with calcium, including orange juices and soy beverages.

Calcium Content of Common Foods

These food sources are high in calcium, though bioavailability varies among sources.

Food Source	Amount	Calcium (mg)
1% milk	1 cup	290
Low-fat fruit yogurt	175 ml	345
Mozzarella cheese (partly skimmed)	1 oz	207
Cheddar cheese	1 oz	204
Low-fat cottage cheese	1 cup	155
Feta cheese	1 oz	140
Frozen yogurt	½ cup	103
Rhubarb (cooked with sugar)	1 cup	348
Figs (dried)	10 figs	140
Collards (boiled, chopped)	1 cup	266
Kale (boiled)	1 cup	179
Okra (boiled)	1 cup	176
Mustard greens (boiled)	1 cup	104
Spinach (boiled, chopped)	1 cup	245
Soybeans (boiled)	1 cup	261
Blackeyed peas (boiled)	1 cup	211
White beans	1 cup	191
Tofu (prepared with calcium sulfate)	¼ block (81 g)	131
Navy beans (boiled)	1 cup	127
Baked beans (canned)	1 cup	127
Great Northern beans (boiled)	1 cup	120
Black turtle beans (boiled)	1 cup	102
Pink salmon (canned)	3 oz	181
Cornbread	1 piece (60 g)	162
Barley	1 cup	158
Cream of Wheat (cooked with water)	1 cup	112
Wheat English muffin	1 muffin	101
Plain instant oatmeal	1 packet (177 g)	99

Adapted from: Dietary Guidelines for Americans, 2005. USDA and U.S. Department of Agriculture, Agricultural Research Service. 2004. USDA Nutrient Database for Standard References, Release 17. Nutrient Data Laboratory. www.nal.usda.gov/fnic/foodcomp

Lactose Intolerance

The enzyme lactase is produced by our body specifically to breakdown a sugar called lactose so that we can absorb it. Lactose is a sugar found in breast milk and in cow's milk. Most children have the proper amount of the enzyme to break down lactose. In many children, as they grow older the amount of the enzyme they produce drops off. The result is that lactose is not broken down. Normal bacteria in the gut are then able to use lactose for energy, and, as a result, they produce gas. The gas they produce can cause bloating and discomfort. More people of Asian and African descent tend to lose their levels of the lactase enzyme sooner than people of European descent.

Saturated Fat in Dairy Products

All dairy products come from whole milk, which contains saturated fat, just like all animal products. Processing and skimming can remove milk-fat. Whole milk can be manufactured into lower-fat milk, cottage cheese, and yogurt. Processing can also remove water content from whole milk, increasing the amount of fat and the energy density of the products as in butter, creams, and cheese.

Because of public demand, dairy producers now offer a wide range of products with a range of different fat content. The percentage of fat and the amount eaten determines the amount of saturated fat eaten. The more total fat in the dairy product, the more saturated fat will be in that product.

Butter Fat Percentage

The fat in dairy products is always labeled on the packaging as the percent of butter fat (% B.F) or percent of milk fat (% M.F). For example, if a cheese has 25% M.F., then in 100 grams of cheese (about four cheese slices), 25% or 25 grams is fat. The remaining 75 grams would be water, protein, and carbohydrate.

Dairy products are typically labeled to show their percentage of butter fat or milk fat: whole (4%), 2%, 1%, 0.5% ('skim'), and 0.1% ('ultra-low fat' or 'fat-free'). Hard cheeses can range in fat from the higher fat varieties, such as cheddar (about 32% M.F.) to the skim milk varieties (about 7% M.F.). Lower-fat cheeses are those labeled 15% M.F. or less.

The lower the percentage of fat, the lower the saturated fat content in products.

FACT

Calcium Need

The recommended amount of total daily calcium:

1–3 years
500 mg/day

4–8 years
800 mg/day

9–18 years
1,300 mg/day

One glass of milk (1 cup) has approximately 300 mg of calcium.

FACT

Lower Lactose Need

The fact that the level of lactase drops in many children as they mature may indicate that milk products are not suitable sources of calcium for all people, especially after childhood and provided nutrition is adequate.

Saturated Fat Content of Common Dairy Foods				
Food	Amount	Energy (Calories)	Total Fat (g)	Saturated Fat (g)
Cheese				
Blue cheese	50 g	100	8.2	5.3
Brie cheese	50 g	95	7.9	4.9
Camembert cheese	50 g	85	6.9	4.3
Cheddar cheese	50 g	114	9.4	6.0
Low-fat cheddar cheese	50 g	49	2.0	1.2
1% Cottage cheese	½ cup	81	1.2	0.7
2% Cottage cheese	½ cup	102	2.2	1.4
Cream cheese (regular)	2 tbsp	99	9.9	6.2
Cream cheese (low-fat)	2 tbsp	65	4.9	3.1
Cream cheese (fat-free)	2 tbsp	27	0.3	0.3
Feta cheese	50 g	75	6.0	4.2
Mozzarella cheese (part-skim)	50 g	72	4.5	2.9
Parmesan cheese (grated)	50 g	122	8.1	4.9
Processed American cheese	50 g	130	4.4	1.9
Processed American cheese (low-fat)	50 g	50	2.0	1.2
Ricotta (part-skim)	50 g	39	2.2	1.4
Swiss	50 g	108	7.9	5.0
Cheez whiz	2 tbsp	91	6.9	4.3
Milk				
Whole milk	1 cup	146	7.9	4.6
2% milk	1 cup	138	4.9	3.0
1% milk	1 cup	102	2.4	1.5
Skim/Non-fat milk	1 cup	83	0.2	0.2

Food	Amount	Energy (Calories)	Total Fat (g)	Saturated Fat (g)
Yogurt/Ice Cream				
Plain yogurt, whole milk	1 cup	149	8.0	5.1
Plain yogurt, low-fat	1 cup	154	3.8	2.5
Plain yogurt, skim	1 cup	137	0.4	0.3
Fruit flavored, low-fat	1 cup	182	2.7	1.7
Fruit flavored, nonfat	1 cup	185	0.5	0.3
Chocolate frozen yogurt	1 cup	221	6.3	4.0
Vanilla frozen yogurt	1 cup	235	8.0	4.9
Vanilla ice cream	1 cup	289	15.8	9.8
Chocolate ice cream	1 cup	285	14.5	9.0
Light chocolate ice cream	1 cup	220	3.7	1.8
Light vanilla ice cream	1 cup	241	5.8	3.8

Adapted from: Dietary Guidelines for Americans, 2005. USDA and U.S. Department of Agriculture, Agricultural Research Service. 2004. USDA Nutrient Database for Standard References, Release 17. Nutrient Data Laboratory. www.nal.usda.gov/fnic/foodcomp

Dairy Food Cautions

The skim and ultra-low-fat varieties have such low saturated fat content that you don't have to worry about them.

Creams

The creams need more caution. Creams (table cream, sour cream) are simply high-fat food with a lot of saturated fat and many calories. They have very little food value. Creams are eaten because we enjoy their flavor or texture, but they should not be considered an essential food — and they should only be eaten in small amounts.

Cheeses

Cheese can be a good source of protein and an additional source of calcium, but it can be very high in saturated fat. Because of the high-fat content in cheese, it is considered an energy dense food with a lot of calories. Many cheese products are now available with reduced amounts of fat with all the protein and calcium of the higher-fat varieties.

Butter

Butter is the highest dairy product on the scale of fat content. Butter is almost entirely fat and water. There is no recommended amount of butter to eat.

Q: **What is the difference between butter and margarine?**

A: Butter and margarine are both simply fats, and, in most cases, they contribute nothing more than extra calories to our diet. The addition of either butter or margarine to foods is unnecessary for health. Many people add butter or margarines to their food out of habit and not necessarily because of taste. If it is not possible to do without butter or margarine, then only small amounts of either should be added to foods.

If you're choosing between using butter or margarine, there are important things to consider. Butter has about the same number of calories and grams of fat as margarine, so there is no difference there. The difference is the type of fat in each. Butter is made from animal milk and is almost entirely saturated fat, which can increase the amount of cholesterol the body produces and contributes additional cholesterol. Margarines are made from plant oils and contain no cholesterol. Some margarines are mostly unsaturated fat, while others are a combination of artificially saturated fat, trans fat, and unsaturated fat.

The consistency of the margarine can tell you a lot about the type of fat used to make it. Saturated fat is solid at room temperature, so, as a general rule, the harder the margarine, the more saturated fat it contains. You may be wondering how margarine can be hard if it is made from plant oils that are liquid at room temperature (the definition of an oil). Most margarines start off as oils that are then processed. The processing is called hydrogenation and results in unsaturated oils becoming harder saturated fat. These are the man-made saturated fats that go into many of the packaged foods we eat, such as cookies and crackers. The non-hydrogenated margarines will contain little or no saturated fat and will be softer. As a general rule, when using margarine go for the softer varieties.

Man-made Saturated Fats

Both man-made and natural saturated fats are linked with cardiovascular disease and should both be limited. Man-made saturated fats are an additional hazard because the hydrogenation process results in the formation of trans fats in addition to saturated fats. Trans fats occur naturally in dairy products, but only in very insignificant amounts. Significant amounts of trans fats can hide is in the margarines located in the dairy section and in processed foods made with hydrogenated oils.

Portions

The available scientific evidence supports the consumption of 1 to 2 servings of dairy products per day. However, calcium can also be obtained from calcium-fortified beverages, such as orange juice and soy beverage or from a calcium supplement.

Q: **How much is one serving of dairy products?**

A: The serving sizes for dairy products were chosen so that they would have approximately the same calcium content as 1 cup (250 ml) of milk, which has 300 milligrams of calcium.

Dairy Product	Servings	Serving size
Milk	1	1 cup (250 ml)
Yogurt	1	¾ cup (175 g)
Block Cheese	1	50 g
Cottage Cheese	1	1 cup
Processed Cheese	1	2 slices (50 g)
Frozen Yogurt	½	½ cup (125 ml)
Pudding	½	½ cup (125 ml)
Ice cream	½	¾ cup (175 ml)

Food Tips

- Be sure that, if buying margarine, you read the label and look for a brand with the lowest amount of saturated fat. Even when low in saturated fat, use as little margarine as possible. It adds unnecessary fat and calories to the diet. If it is used for oiling a pan during cooking, consider switching to an oil spray instead.

- Avoid any margarine that has the words "hydrogenated" or "partially-hydrogenated" because these will have trans fats. As a general rule, harder margarines have more man-made saturated fat, as well as also have more trans fats. When choosing margarine, choose varieties labeled with the claim "Low in saturated fat," which means it has less than 2 grams of saturated and trans fat.

- Use 1% or 2% evaporated milk as a substitute for real cream in puddings, sauces, and casseroles.

- Try using applesauce or pureed prunes as a substitute for oil or butter in baked goods.

- Use low-fat chicken broth for flavoring in mashed potatoes instead of butter or cream.

- Consider calcium-fortified soy beverages as a non-dairy source of calcium.

- Fat-free and low-fat yogurt can be used for shakes, dips, and snacks.

CHAPTER 6

Healthy Weight Food Choices

Part 2: Processed and Preserved Foods

 FACT

Advertising Food

Food manufacturers, retailers, and food services spent $11 billion in 1997 on mass media advertising. In the same year, the USDA (United States Department of Agriculture) spent $333.3 million on nutrition education, evaluation and demonstration — only 3% of what the food industry spent.

Thanks to agricultural and technological developments over the past century, hunger and starvation are now rare among North Americans, even during the winter season. We have developed means to preserve fresh food by processing and packaging it. There is now a constant supply of high calorie, energy dense foods. However, these foods have become so popular that they are displacing fresh whole food, even when it is available.

We are easily convinced to consume these processed and preserved foods and many of us do so in large quantities. The producers make the taste appealing and use advertising to promote their latest processed food invention. In addition, these foods are convenient. We tend to lead very busy lifestyles, where time spent preparing wholesome food is sacrificed for more time spent at work or in other activities. For many who have limited time for preparing food, convenience of food has become a necessity.

Because of these appeals, we seem to be losing touch with the signals our body sends about our nutritional needs. Instead, we ignore signs of overweight, opting for foods that will only worsen our health.

Processed and preserved foods can be high in calories and low in nutrients. We often find ourselves craving high fat and/or high sugar food and the food industry readily responds to our demands by ensuring these foods are always available and at a lesser cost than more nutritious alternatives. If we are going to eat processed foods and maintain some level of health, we have to reconnect with our body's actual food needs and teach ourselves healthy eating behavior. The only way we can make smart food choices among the processed and packaged foods we eat is to understand food nutrition labels.

CASE STUDY Anne's Family

A Setback and Recovery

Several days over the past week, Cody had brought back home significant amounts of the lunch that he prepared every morning. "Why don't you finish your lunch?" Anne asked. "I'm just not that hungry," shrugged Cody. "That's because he buys chips and candy every day," Mark chimed in. Cody gave Mark a cold stare. "Is that true, Cody?" Bill asked. "Sometimes," Cody whispered. Bill was starting to get angry, and Cody was starting to get nervous. "Don't you know that those things are only for treats, not for every day?" Bill demanded. "I thought we had an agreement." "It's hard!" Cody cried. "Do you want me to take away your allowance?" Bill exclaimed. He had to cool off. "I can't believe you can buy that stuff right in the schools these days," he muttered as he walked away.

Cody was crying, and Mark was acting smug. "Mark, it isn't nice to tattle on your brother, and Cody, we need to work this out," Anne said. They talked for a while. Cody agreed that he had been doing so well, and that the weight he had lost made him feel proud. He didn't want to mess things up, but it was hard when the other kids were buying the stuff. Anne worked out a plan in which Cody would stop buying things on his own at the school, and that they would go to the grocery store and see if they could find something healthier that he liked that he could take in his lunch for a treat. That evening Anne and Bill agreed that it was time to meet with Cody's principal and discuss their concerns about junk food being sold in the school.

continued on page 185

Food Nutrition Labels

If we only ate fresh unprocessed foods and made fruit, vegetables, whole grains, and legumes the largest portion of our diet, there would be little need to understand the nutrition label. If we need to supplement our diet with processed and packaged foods, we need to learn to read nutrition labels.

Many food companies compete for our attention and our dollars. If they cannot keep us buying their products, they will go out of business. Unfortunately, some companies have to walk the fine line between making a profit and providing nutritious food at whatever the cost. The information provided on the packaging of food can have a major impact on whether or not we purchase a product.

In the past, some companies have resorted to questionable advertising methods to encourage selection of their products. Government regulatory agencies are beginning to restrict these practices more and more. Still, a great deal of responsibility is left in the hands of the consumer. By learning how to read labels, you can make better choices when selecting processed and packaged food.

When making decisions about what processed foods to buy, there are two reasons why reading the food label is very important:

1. Because we allow the food industry to make our food for us, we don't always know what ingredients they are using without reading the label.

2. Because foods that are high in calories and low in nutrients are often easier and less expensive to process and preserve, the food industry may try to encourage us to buy more and eat more of these foods.

By reading food labels, we can determine which processed foods are best and what amounts are appropriate for achieving a healthy weight and maintaining good health. We are going to take you through the process of making smart nutritional choices for your child and we will simplify it for you.

Four Food Label Facts

Learning to read food labels is not difficult. Once you have studied them, you can pick out the four most important facts.

1. Nutrient Content Claims: These claims tell you about one specific nutrient, for example, sodium, fat, or sugar content.

2. Health Claims: These claims tell you how the food may affect your health.

3. Ingredients List: This important list tells you what ingredients are in the packaged food.

4. Nutrition Fact Label: These labels give you information on the number of calories and the amount of 13 different nutrients for a specific serving size of the food.

For more information on food labels, contact the Nutrition Education and Labeling Centre (www.healthyeatingisinstore.ca) and the United States Food and Drug Administration (FDA) Center for Food Safety and Applied Nutrition (www.cfsan.fda.gov).

Nutrient Content Claims

Nutrient content claims were designed to help us determine specific information about fat, sugar, salt, cholesterol, and calories in packaged food at a glance. When reading these claims, we have to be careful about their meaning. Sometimes, they can give us a false sense of the nutritive value of the foods we are buying. Occasionally, food manufacturers may also take advantage of the Nutrition Labeling System for their profit.

For example, some products have always been low in carbohydrates. However, with the low carbohydrate craze, manufacturers are taking advantage of this by producing "low-carb" labeling. Suddenly, foods that are naturally low in carbohydrate become avoided only because they haven't been labeled as such.

A food that is predominantly made of sugar or fat may be a good source of a vitamin. The label may say "an excellent source" of the vitamin. However, the high sugar and fat content may outweigh the benefit of that vitamin (which often can be obtained by eating a small amount of fruit or vegetables). The fact that the label has a positive message about the vitamin may be the deciding factor convincing you to buy it even when it is not the healthiest option.

The food industry may use these claims to increase the sale of their product in other ways. For example, since the recommendations that North Americans should reduce their fat intake, the number of so-called low-fat products that have been introduced to the market has skyrocketed. The low-fat claim may convince you that this product is okay to eat when trying to keep fat limited in the diet. The problem is that often these foods leave off the label claim that says "high in sugar," which means that the product may actually have *more* calories than the regular fat variety. You may also be inclined to eat more of a low-fat product in one sitting, which can defeat the whole purpose of buying it in the first place. We know that all excess calories we consume are stored as fat, regardless of whether they came from fat, carbohydrate, or protein.

> ## Food Warning!
> Watch out for claims such as "95% fat-free" — these foods are still 5% fat! Some manufacturers use this statement instead of 5% fat because it makes the product appear lower in fat.

Key to Nutrient Content Claims

Food labels are written to give us a greater sense of comfort about choosing the product. However, we need to question these claims in the context of our knowledge of food energy and nutrition.

Fat Content Claims

The following are a list of the types of fat content claims you will find on food labels. These claims all appeal to our fear of consuming fat.

Claim	Meaning
Fat-free	0.5 grams of fat per serving
Low-fat	3 grams or less total fat per 100 gram serving. This may appear on the package as "97% (or more) fat free" or "3% (or less) fat "
Reduced fat	Product has 25% less fat than the same regular brand
Light	Product has 50% less fat than the same regular brand
Low saturated fat	2 grams or less per serving
Low cholesterol	20 milligrams or less per serving and low in saturated fat

Cautions

1. Lower fat, higher calories: If comparing a reduced fat cookie (25% less fat) with the regular brand, unless you read the Nutrition Fact Label, you won't know that:

- Lower-fat products can have the same number of calories as the regular version.
- Lower-fat products may have more sugar added to make up for missing fat.

Sometimes, the lower-fat products actually contain even more calories than the regular version. Remember, the Positive Energy Rule means that no matter whether the calories come from fat or extra sugar, the excess are always stored as body fat.

2. Lower fat, lower filling: Studies show that the fat content of our food can affect how full we feel after eating the food and for how long. In one study, participants either ate fat-free muffins or muffins made with oil. Both kinds of muffins had the same amount of energy (calories) but the participants eating the fat-free muffins felt less full afterward and more hungry. The participants eating the low-fat muffins didn't eat any fewer calories over the day. When considering lower fat options it is important to consider the following:

- Lower-fat processed foods and baked goods may not make you feel full and make you feel more hungry, which can lead to overeating.
- Eating lower-fat processed foods does not necessarily lower the number of calories eaten in a day, making them ineffective for losing body fat

When eating lower-fat processed food, we may be consuming the exact same amount of calories (as mentioned above), we may not feel as full and this may lead us to overeat or to eat again sooner than we normally would. In both cases, we could end up eating more calories and the Positive Energy Rule would apply.

3. Low in saturated fat, high in total fat: It is important that we try to avoid saturated fat in our diet because it is linked to cardiovascular disease. Just because a product claims to be low in saturated fat does not mean, however, that it is a low-fat product. It may have a large amount of unsaturated fat and sugar, which both can be a source of excessive calories.

4. Cholesterol and saturated fat: Saturated fat in the diet has a much greater effect on our blood cholesterol levels than the cholesterol in the foods we eat. When the amount of saturated fat in the diet is kept low, cholesterol levels in the diet will also be low. Food products that are made from plant sources only will always be cholesterol free, and in these cases, the label "cholesterol free" is stating the obvious and is likely designed to encourage us to buy that product because we feel that it is healthier.

> **Food Warning!**
> Beware of nutrient content claims because they are sometimes related to a serving size much smaller than what a person would normally eat.

Q: **Based on this information and these cautions, should I choose regular or low-fat versions of processed foods?**

A: Choose the product lower in saturated fat but bear in mind that it should *not* be consumed in higher quantities. Also, look for the product with more fiber and less calories and no trans fat.

Calorie Content Claims

Claim	*Meaning*
Calorie-free	Fewer than 5 Calories per serving
Calorie reduced	50% or fewer calories compared with the regular version
Low calorie	40 Calories or less per serving

Cautions

These claims encourage us to buy the products bearing them when we are attempting to limit our calorie intake to a healthy level. Remember, a normal serving of lower-calorie foods must be eaten to decrease the number of calories eaten. This may seem simple and obvious, but many people will overeat foods when they believe that they are low-calorie. In fact, they will often eat much more of those foods than they normally would and increase the number of calories eaten above the amount of the regular calorie version.

Sodium Content Claims

Claim	*Meaning*
Low-sodium	140 mg or less sodium per serving

Caution

Salt (sodium) is found in large amounts in many processed foods. Because of this, choosing lower-salt versions of products is always a healthier choice.

Sugar Content Claims

Claim	*Meaning*
Unsweetened	Only naturally occurring sugars are present
No sugar added	Naturally occurring sugars are still present

Caution

These claims mean that no sugar was added to the product. You must be careful because these foods can still have a large amount of naturally occurring sugar. In fact, adding concentrated fruit juice (with a concentrated amount of sugar) still qualifies the product to bear these claims, even though, technically, sugar has been added.

Food Warning!

Be aware that sometimes health claims can give you a sense of comfort that encourage you to buy more of these products. Be especially cautious when these labels appear on more processed foods. Health claims are not a valid excuse to overeat any foods.

Health Claims

Health claims point to a single ingredient as being shown to help prevent a disease.

Such claims may state, for example, that "Development of cancer depends on many factors. A diet low in total fat may reduce the risk of some cancers."

Scientists and consumers are always looking for the magic bullet that will prevent heart disease, diabetes, cancer, and other health problems. Even though studies may show that a specific vitamin, mineral, spice, or phytochemical can lead to a reduction in a specific disease, it is unwise to take large amounts of that one nutrient. Most often, it is the overall diet that is most influential in determining health, not the over-consumption of just one food. Avoid the temptation of buying one food containing that ingredient and instead go for variety.

Ingredients Lists

The ingredient list is extremely important because, legally, it must reveal all the specific ingredients (healthy and unhealthy) in the product. This is especially helpful for people with allergies. The ingredients list can also benefit consumers because they can see if products have less healthy ingredients.

Q: How do I read the ingredients list?

A: When we read the ingredients list, we will look for nutrients and additives not mentioned directly on the Nutrition Fact Label. The ingredients are ranked according to the amount in the product. The first few ingredients in the list make up the largest amount in the food product. For example, most cookies would likely contain a lot of enriched flour (which acts like sugar in our body), a lot of glucose or sugar (which goes straight from our stomach into our bloodstream), and a lot of partially-hydrogenated vegetable (which means saturated fat and trans fat).

Cautions

You will need to be aware of how certain ingredients are named in the ingredients list to help you make better choices.

Saturated Fat

Natural sources of saturated fat are present when the following ingredients are listed: butter, coconut or coconut oil, palm or palm kernel oil, cocoa butter, powdered whole milk solids, tallow or beef fat, lard, suet, chicken fat, and bacon fat.

Man-made Saturated Fat

Some foods are normally low in saturated fat but become more saturated during processing. Key words to look for on a label are hydrogenated or partially hydrogenated and shortening. Hydrogenation is a process food manufacturers use to turn liquid oil into a solid form, making it more saturated.

Trans Fats

The same hydrogenation process used to convert unsaturated fat into saturated fat also produces trans fat. Manufacturers use hydrogenated oils for several reasons. They are more solid, which may give a more enjoyable texture to the product; they have a higher melting point, so they can be used for frying at higher temperatures (as in fast-food French fries, chicken, fish); and they have a longer shelf life before spoilage, which is important for decreasing the costs and increasing the profits from these products.

Hydrogenated oils were brought into the market around the time that saturated fats were getting a bad rap. Before the saturated fat scare, coconut oil, palm oil, and cocoa butter – all high in saturated fats — were commonly used in processed food recipes. The food industry was partially responding to a consumer demand for what was thought to be a healthier alternative to these saturated fats. However, it was the wrong move.

Food Warning!

Man-made saturated fat and the resulting trans fats should be phased out of our diet. Consider that whenever we eat any products with trans fat, we are putting ourselves at increased risk for disease. Trans fat should be completely avoided. By the year 2006, all Nutrition Fact panels on packaged food in North America will have to state the amount of trans fat present. Until then, it is up to the consumer to identify and avoid products containing them.

✔ FACT • Trans Fats and Disease

Studies indicate that consumption of trans fat is associated with chronic diseases, such as heart disease, cancer, and diabetes. Scientists also worry that they may have a negative effect on our immune system and on reproduction. A large Harvard University study of nurses found that eating less saturated and trans fats, not unsaturated fats, was important for decreasing cardiovascular disease.

Trans fats are more dangerous to our health than satu-rated fats. In the body, trans fats act like saturated fat in that they increase the 'bad' LDL (low density lipoprotein) choles-terol in the blood. Another major problem with trans fat is that our body was not designed with the right enzymes to handle these man-made fats properly.

Trans Fats by Food Groups

The major dietary sources of trans fats are listed here in decreasing order. Processed foods and oils provide approximately 80% of trans fats in the diet, while 20% occur naturally in food from animal sources. Trans fat content of certain processed foods has changed and is likely to continue to change as the industry reformulates products.

Food Group	Contribution (percent of total trans fats consumed)
Baked goods (cakes, cookies, crackers, pies, bread, etc.)	40
Animal products	21
Margarine	17
Fried potatoes	8
Potato chips, corn chips, popcorn	5
Household shortening	4
Other (candy, breakfast cereal, etc.)	5

Adapted from Federal Register notice. *Food Labeling; Trans Fatty Acids in Nutrition Labeling; Consumer Research To Consider Nutrient Content and Health Claims and Possible Footnote or Disclosure Statements; Final Rule and Proposed Rule.* Vol. 68, No. 133, p. 41433-41506, July 11, 2003. Data collected 1994-1996.

Q: What foods contain the most trans fats?

A: Most of the trans fats we eat will come from processed foods. These include commercial baked goods, fried foods, margarine, shortening, and packaged foods, such as cakes, cookies, corn chips, crackers, donuts, chips, and French fries. Many fast food restaurants use hydrogenated fats in their deep fryers, which are then transferred to the foods fried in them.

Sugars and Sugar Alcohols
Both sugars and sugar alcohols add extra calories to food products. Sugars are present whenever ingredients ending in 'ose' are listed in the ingredients list, such as: fructose, high fructose corn syrup, sucrose, maltose, lactose, galactose, dextrose. They are also present when these other ingredients are listed: honey, liquid sugar, invert sugar, liquid invert sugar, syrup, dextrin, corn syrup solids, molasses, and syrup.

Sugar alcohols are present whenever ingredients ending in 'ol' are listed in the ingredients list, such as: lacitol, mannitol, maltitol, sorbitol, xylitol, and isomalt

Salt
Sodium (salt) is present whenever the following are listed in the ingredients list: monosodium glutamate, baking powder, baking soda, sodium alginate, sodium benzoate, sodium hydroxide, sodium propionate, sodium bisulfate, brine, garlic salt, onion salt, celery salt, and soy sauce.

Nutrition Facts Labels

Nutrition Facts labels are intended to inform you about the nutritive value of the food so that you can make smarter and healthier food choices. Using information on these labels will ensure that you and your family are getting the right amount of calories, vitamins, minerals, and fiber from the food you buy. The information will also help you avoid excess fat and sugar. The Nutrition Facts label allows you to be more educated about the food you eat.

There are several very important items listed in the Nutrition Facts label and we will explain each of these in the order they appear:

1. Serving Size (Portion Size)
The first and most important thing to notice is the serving size stated on the Nutrition Facts label. There are several ways that the serving size of packaged food is described and measured, depending on whether the food is individually wrapped into predetermined portions, whether the food is a liquid or a solid, and whether it is eaten as a whole item or poured. You will find measurements such as "package," "# of items," cup, milliliters (ml), ounces (oz), and grams (g).

Everything else you read on the fact label is based on one serving. For example, a serving size for breakfast cereal may be 1 cup (30 grams). When the food label lists the number of calories in the cereal, it is listing the number of calories in 1 cup (1 serving) of the cereal. When the food label lists the amount of sugars or vitamins in the food, it is also listing the amount in 1 cup of the cereal. That means that if you tend to eat more than this amount, you need to take the extra amount into consideration.

Serving Size Cautions
The size of a serving specified on labels is determined by the food manufacturers. It is usually a typical amount eaten, but sometimes it is a lot smaller or a lot larger. Because of this, it should not be seen as the recommended amount that should be eaten.

In fact, the serving size listed may be larger than what nutritionists and dietitians recommend for healthy serving sizes. The increase in portion sizes and the 'super-size' phenomenon has changed what North Americans think of as a normal portion. You may believe that the listed serving size is normal when it is actually much too large. The serving size may seem small when it is actually a more appropriate amount.

With individually wrapped food items, sometimes the size of the item is actually larger than the listed serving size. When servings are individually wrapped, people are more likely to eat the entire item, even if they not hungry for that amount. You will need to bear in mind that by eating the whole item, you may be eating more than one serving.

> **Food Warning!**
> Occasionally, food companies use an unrealistically small portion size. The effect of this is that it reduces the apparent amount of sugar and fat per serving. However, the typical amount eaten of these foods will be many servings, with much more sugar and fat.

2. Calories
It is important to notice the number of calories for the specific serving size listed. If more than a serving is eaten normally, then more calories are being eaten than what is listed. Often children and adults consume more than the serving size listed on the label.

Food manufactures may list the portion size as "one cookie," for example. This means that the number of calories, amount of fat and sugar, and all other values on the label will appear low because they only refer to one small cookie. When it comes to less nutritious food, this may convince you to buy more because it appears to be a low-calorie, low-fat, or low-sugar option. The problem with this is that often the consumer (your child) may eat five or six of those cookies in one sitting. Remember that you must multiply the number of calories and amount of fat and sugar listed on the label by five or six times (the number of cookies).

Finally, remember that a calorie is a calorie whether it comes from fat, protein, or carbohydrate. It is the number of calories consumed, not the type of food, that determines if we will store calories as body fat.

Calories from Fat

If the label does not specifically list the number of calories from fat, there is an easy way to figure it out. Just add zero after the number of grams of fat listed on the label. For example, if the label lists 10 grams of fat per serving, adding zero means 100. This means that there are 100 Calories from fat. The reason this works is because each gram of fat has 9 Calories. We are simply rounding 9 Calories up to an even 10 Calories and multiplying by the total number of grams of fat in the serving. Then, look again at the total calories in one serving. If the total calories per serving is 200 Calories, and 100 Calories is coming from fat, that means that half (50%) of the calories are from fat. This is much higher than the recommended 35%.

3. Nutrients

The Nutrition Facts label gives information about the following nutrients.

Fat

Often the different types of fat are listed here. With processed food, the goal is to keep saturated fat to a minimum. If only the total fat is listed on less healthy food choices, it may be because the listing of the amount of saturated and trans fats in the product would discourage you from buying it.

Cholesterol

Because the body (the liver) makes most of the cholesterol we need, very little is required from the diet. Also, too much cholesterol in the blood can lead to heart disease and stroke down the road. Because cholesterol is present in some of the natural foods we eat, such as eggs, poultry, and meat, aim to avoid cholesterol in packaged food. Cholesterol recommendations for children over the age of 2 are the same as for adults: no more than 300 milligrams per day.

Food Warning!

Foods claiming to be "low cholesterol" on the labels may still be high in fat. High intake of saturated fat is a large contributor to high blood cholesterol.

Q: **What does Recommended Dietary Allowance (RDA) mean?**

A: Recommended Dietary Allowances are the nutrient intake recommendations from the Institute of Medicine, an arm of the American Academy of Sciences. RDAs are safe levels of intake for essential nutrients, based on current scientific knowledge. They are set to meet the known nutrient needs of practically all healthy people. RDAs have been around and updated regularly for more than 50 years. RDAs are gradually being replaced by revised guidelines called Dietary Reference Intakes or DRIs, a collaboration between Canadian and American health authorities. DRIs are being developed for vitamins and minerals that currently have no RDAs.

Sodium

Packaged and processed foods often have high sodium content used for flavor and to preserve the food. Food manufacturers often add sodium even to sweet foods to make you want to eat more. Notice that often after eating something sweet, you crave something salty and vice versa. Sodium is important for proper fluid levels in the body, but too much sodium may be harmful. The high level of sodium in the diet is predominately a result of processed food intake and not salt added to food in the home.

Carbohydrate

Total carbohydrate includes all complex carbohydrates (starches), simple carbohydrates (sugars), and the non-digestible carbohydrates (fiber). Often the sugars and fiber content are listed separately also.

Fiber

Fiber is important for your family's health. It is recommended that children get the equivalent of their Age + 5 in grams of fiber per day. Look for products with the nutritional claims: "source of dietary fiber" (2 to 4 grams), "high source of dietary fiber" (4 to 6 grams), "very high source of fiber" (6 grams or more).

To find good sources of fiber in the ingredients list, look for the following ingredients: 100% whole wheat flour, wheat bran, oat bran, and corn bran.

 FACT

Salt Limits
The American Heart Association recommends that for every 1000 Calories consumed, sodium intake should be 1000 milligrams (½ teaspoon) and should not exceed the 3000 milligram limit. The average intake among North Americans is higher than recommended.

Sugars

Often these represent the simple refined sugars added to processed and packaged foods and provide very little nutritional value. Look to buy products that have very low amounts of the simple sugars.

✔ FACT • Sugar Limits

The USDA recommends consuming less than 40 grams (10 teaspoons) of sugar per day (about 1 can of pop/soda). Choose food products with less than 15 grams of sugars per serving (the lower the better). Remember, that eating more than a serving means that more sugar is being eaten. Also, limit adding additional sugar to foods. Each teaspoon of sugar is 4 grams.

Percentage of recommended daily limit on added sugar (40 grams, 10 teaspoons)

1 can of pop/soda	100%
1 cup regular ice cream	60%
1 cup sweetened yogurt	70%
1 cup sweet breakfast cereal	30%
1 candy bar	60%

Protein

Most of the important protein in your child's diet should be coming from more whole sources of food and not processed foods. In general, it isn't necessary to concern yourself with the protein levels in processed foods. It is recommended that protein make up between 10% and 20% of our daily calorie intake.

Vitamins

At the very least, you will find the vitamins A and C listed on food labels because manufacturers realize that these vitamins may be lacking in our diets since fruit and vegetable consumption is low.

Minerals

At the very least, you will find the minerals calcium and iron listed on food labels. A lack of these minerals can lead to health complications.

Q: What is the % Daily Value?

A: The % Daily Value tells you how much of the daily recommended amount for each nutrient is provided by one serving. The recommended amount is based on eating a 2000-Calorie diet. Very active people who need more than 2000 Calories per day will need to get more than the % Daily Value listed. Inactive people who need less than 2000 Calories per day will not need to get all of the % Daily Value listed.

Using the % Daily Value, you can determine if there is a small amount or large amount of the specific nutrient in the food. For example, a low number, such as 5% or less for % Daily Value indicates that there is a small amount of that nutrient in the serving. A high number, such as 20% or greater, indicates that there is a large amount.

Eating mostly fresh, unprocessed foods will provide all the essential nutrients your child needs to be healthy. When time constraints or convenience make packaged foods necessary choices, the % Daily Value rating can be helpful.

The % Daily Values are additive, that is, if one serving of food contains a 25% Daily Value for vitamin A and a serving of another food contains a 10% Daily Value for vitamin A, then eating both of these servings would give you 25+10 = 35% of the recommended Daily Value for vitamin A.

% Daily Value Goals

Vitamins	Get 100%		Saturated fat	Get no more than 100%
Minerals	Get 100%		Cholesterol	Get no more than 100%
Fiber	Get 100%		Sodium	Get no more than 100%

To help accomplish these goals

1. Choose foods with a high % Daily Values for these key nutrients:
- Fiber   • Vitamin A   • Vitamin C   • Calcium   • Iron

2. Choose foods with a low % Daily Value for these nutrients:
- Saturated Fat   • Cholesterol   • Sodium

A special note about calcium: the recommendations are that children ages 4 to 8 should get a total of 80% when adding the % Daily Values for calcium. For children ages 9 to 18, extra calcium is recommended to maximize their bone growth, and 130% is recommended when adding up the % Daily Values.

Guidelines for Buying Processed Food

Homemade

Whenever possible, prepare at home the food that you would normally buy packaged. Even if they are once in a while foods like cookies or cakes, when made at home you'll have control over the quality and amount of ingredients. You won't need preservatives or trans fat containing ingredients.

Read Before You Buy

Always read nutrition labels to discover what is in the food that you are buying. Processed food is not always intended to be a healthy option.

Creamy Labels

Foods that advertise their creamy nature often are high in saturated fat. Keep these creamier foods to a minimum to reduce saturated fat.

Five Good Reasons to Limit Processed Foods

1. Nutrition

Processed foods may contain lots of added sugar and salt, and often contain saturated fats. These foods are high in calories and are low in nutrients.

2. Mystery Ingredients

They may have ingredients with names that are difficult to pronounce, which give the product its texture, color, and flavor.

3. Overconsumption

Millions of dollars are spent to design processed foods that satisfy, yet keep people coming back for more. For example, reducing the flavorings in some foods can mean that you are not totally satisfied by only a small amount.

4. Trans Fats

Processed foods may be made with hydrogenated or partially hydrogenated oils.

5. Artificial Flavors and Colors

Both "natural flavor" and "artificial flavor" are man-made additives that give processed food most of its taste. They are used for several reasons. Canning, freezing, and dehydrating techniques used to process food destroy most of its natural flavor. In addition, the careful manipulation of food flavor can have an impact on the amount of that food we eat and on cravings.

Artificial colors are used to make processed food more appealing to us. Brightly colored foods often seem to taste better than bland-looking foods.

Mystery Meat

The quality of meat in processed foods is very difficult to determine after it has been ground up, mashed, and mixed with sugar, salt, spices, and coloring agents. The meat fillings in many packaged foods may be from poorer quality, higher fat cuts of meat that might not sell as regular cuts in the meat section. They can be high in saturated fat. When possible, choose to buy fresh meat of any kind from a trusted source.

Enriched Advertising

The word 'Enriched' may give you a sense of quality about the food. 'Enriched wheat flour' is simply white flour that has some of the vitamins added back that were lost in making the whole grain into processed white flour. Don't be fooled into believing that enriched wheat flour indicates a healthier choice. Multigrain in the name of a product doesn't mean whole wheat either! Simply adding a few whole grains to the top of a loaf of bread might be all it takes to give the product a 'multigrain' name. Be sure to check the ingredients list to find out if it is really a whole grain product.

Breading with Calories

Some meat entrées in the frozen food section are breaded. When these foods are breaded, extra calories are being added (the flour in the breading) and from the frying process that cooks the meat with the breading before it is frozen for you to buy. Cutting back on breaded foods is a good way to reduce calories and often fat.

 FACT

Pass on Pastry

Processed food pastries or frozen entrées, including those with meat inside pastry will have high levels of saturated fat. Pastry foods should be kept to a minimum when trying to reduce saturated fat and excess calories.

Cooking Oils

Using oils that are unsaturated instead of saturated fats, such as butter, lard, or vegetable shortening, is a healthier option. Be aware that all oils are 100% fat. When the label on cooking oils says "light" it is only referring to the color or flavor of the oil. There is no such thing as a lower-fat oil.

The method you use to cook food and the amount of oil you use can have a major impact on the number of calories in the meal. Choosing cooking oils that are higher in monounsaturated fat, such as olive oil, are healthier options, but do not use excessive amounts.

Food Tips

- Use low-fat cooking methods instead of frying. These include baking, broiling, boiling, grilling, microwaving, poaching, roasting, and steaming.

- Use cooking oil sprays to replace margarine or oil as a lubricant.

Percentages of Some Specific Types of Fat in Common Oils and fats

Oils	Saturated	Monounsaturated	Polyunsaturated	Trans
Canola	7	58	29	0
Safflower	9	12	74	0
Sunflower	10	20	66	0
Corn	13	24	60	0
Olive	13	72	8	0
Soybean	16	44	37	0
Peanut	17	49	32	0
Palm	50	37	10	0
Coconut	87	6	2	0
Cooking Fats				
Shortening	22	29	29	18
Lard	39	44	11	1
Butter	60	26	5	5
Margarine/Spreads				
70% Soybean Oil, Stick	18	2	29	23
67% Corn and Soybean Oil Spread, Tub	16	27	44	11
48% Soybean Oil Spread, Tub	17	24	49	8
60% Sunflower, Soybean, and Canola Oil Spread, Tub	18	22	54	5

Values expressed as percent of total fat. Data comes from analyses at Harvard School of Public Health Lipid Laboratory and USDA publications. www.hsph.harvard.edu/nutritionsource/fats.html

CASE STUDY Anne's Family

School Food

As Anne and Bill walked into the school's main entrance, they noticed the panel of vending machines, full of soft drinks, chips, candy, and chocolate bars. "What next? A cigarette machine?" Bill sniped. There was a poster on the wall announcing "Pizza Lunch Day every Thursday."

They were escorted into the principal's office, where Mr. MacLean introduced himself. Anne and Bill explained the health situation with Cody and how they felt it was not appropriate to be promoting and selling junk food in a school. Mr. MacLean explained that the school received significant revenue from contracts they had with these companies, and that revenue had become essential in keeping many of the school's programs going. He agreed that he felt very ambivalent about it, but the school board had promoted and endorsed it. The vending machines were there to stay.

Bill wasn't impressed, but Anne felt more optimistic. She suggested that maybe they could have some healthier alternatives offered in the vending machines, like water and unsweetened juices, and low-fat pretzels, for example. They could also make those items more marketable by raising the prices of the less ideal items in order to be able to lower the prices for the healthier alternatives. She suggested that they move the vending machines out of a high-traffic area, and definitely far away from where the kids ate their lunch.

Mr. MacLean thought that those were some great suggestions. He asked Anne and Bill if they would like to help organize a combined student, teacher, and parent group that might look at ways to make the school healthier. One small battle won, thought Anne to herself.

continued on page 178

Salad Dressings

Oil-based salad dressings can turn a nutritious, low-calorie salad into a high-fat, high-calorie meal. In fact, the addition of dressings to salads at fast-food restaurants can often raise the fat and calories higher than the highest fat burger meal sold. "Low calorie" or "light" dressing should be used when trying to reduce the amount of fat and number of calories in the diet. Keep the amount of dressing to a minimum.

Food Tips

- Make sure a 1-tablespoon serving of salad dressing has no more than 2 grams of saturated fat.

- The creamier looking dressings tend to be higher in saturated fat and overall fat.

- A light salad before a meal is a great way to achieve the recommended daily number of servings of vegetables.

Condiments, Sauces, Spreads, and Dips

Condiments and Sauces

Mustards, ketchup, and relishes are generally fat-free, but not all condiments are low in calories. In the case of mustard and relish, they are relatively low in calories and a very large amount would have to be eaten to have a significant effect on calorie intake. Ketchup and many other sauces, such as sweet and sour sauce and barbeque sauce, have loads of added sugar. Eating ketchup or these other sauces does not become a problem when small amounts are used. When larger amounts are used, they can contribute a considerable amount of calories to a meal without providing many nutrients. Sometimes sauces can be extremely high in fat and saturated fat, too. This is especially the case with creamy sauces, such as those used with pasta. Tomato-based sauces tend to have almost no fat. Soy sauces should be used in moderation because they tend to be high in salt.

Food Tips

- Choose salsa or low-fat hummus as dips instead of creamy dips.

- Use citrus juices, herbs, and spices to add flavor to food without adding fat.

- Decrease the amount of cream and butter sauces used to lower the amount of saturated fat in the diet.

- Make dips, spreads or sauces at home to control the amount and quality of ingredients.

Spreads and Dips

It is very difficult to account for all the different spreads and dips available in the grocery stores today. The varieties of products also have various sugar and fat content, with some having extremely high-fat content. As a general rule, products with dairy products (milk or cream) or whole eggs will have more saturated fat and should be limited. Spreads made with non-hydrogenated unsaturated oils, such as olive oil or nut spreads, are better choices.

Frozen Foods

Frozen Meals

There are times when home-cooked meals are just not possible and frozen meals become the best option for you. When you buy these foods, you will have to use your nutrition label reading skills to make healthier choices. Extra time spent finding healthy frozen meals is time well spent.

Frozen entrées often contain 'mystery' meat. It is often difficult to determine the quality of the meat, and the saturated fat content may be very high. Frozen entrées made with pastries will often have very high amounts of saturated fats, so avoid these options when you're looking for frozen meals.

Food Tips

- Freezing your produce at home is also an option to keep food around longer. You'll need to experiment with different packaging techniques so that when thawed, the food still has a texture you enjoy.

- When buying frozen dinners, choose entrées with a total of 10 or less grams of fat.

- Choosing frozen meals made with quality lean meat is a better option when trying to keep saturated fat to a minimum.

- Limit foods made with lots of dairy, such as creams and cheeses, because they are often high in saturated fats. Breaded and fried foods will also have a lot of extra fat and calories without additional nutritional value.

- When buying frozen burgers, choose lower-fat versions, such as extra-lean or lean beef, sirloin, veggie, chicken, or turkey. Remember, that doesn't mean eating more.

- Choose extra-lean entrées using boneless skinless chicken breast.

Soups

Soups can make great snacks or can even be the main course. However, canned soups can be high in salt content with poorer quality meat. Just like some of the meat in frozen entrées, the meat in soups may contain a significant amount of saturated fat.

Soups made with dairy products will also tend to be higher in saturated fats and should be limited when trying to reduce saturated fat intake. These include cream of mushroom and cream of broccoli.

Food Tips

- When buying canned vegetable soups, the main thing to look out for is the salt content, which can quite high compared with soups made at home from scratch. When possible, select reduced salt varieties.

- Buy vegetable-based soups and add fresh vegetables and freshly cooked meat afterward.

- If you are making soups and stews using animal products or even when they are store bought, cooling them in the fridge will solidify the saturated fat and allow you to remove it from the top before re-heating it.

Breakfast Foods and Cereals

Cereals can contain plenty of nutrients and can be quite filling, especially when they are made with whole grains. *The European Journal of Clinical Nutrition* reported that eating cereal for breakfast regularly can lead to reduced intake of total and saturated fat in the daily diet and consequently to a reduction in cholesterol levels.

Even though they may have lots of vitamins and minerals, breakfast cereals should not be eaten in very large quantities. Along with those extra nutrients also come a lot of calories. They may not be great as snack foods.

Sugar

Most breakfast cereals have added sugar, so you want to choose those with the least amount added.

Whole Grains

Eating whole-grain, but not refined-grain, breakfast cereal intake has been shown to decrease the risk of heart disease. Whole grains also fill you up faster because they're high in fiber.

Saturated Fat

Cereals that contain coconut and granola often contain saturated fat, so choose low-fat versions of these. Completely avoid cereals that include trans fat or "partially hydrogenated oil."

Cereal Bars

Some cereal bars can be low in fat and even fortified with vitamins, but often they are low in whole grains and fiber. They are just fortified candy bars. Remember that eating white flour or other refined grains is just like eating pure sugar.

Portions

Be aware of serving sizes with cereal because they are determined by weight. Usually 30 grams of cereal is considered 1 serving. This can be as much as 1 cup for some cereals and as little as ⅓ cup for others.

Food Warning!

Don't be fooled by nutrient claims. Even if a cereal boasts "High Fiber," "Excellent Source of Calcium," or "Organic," it still may contain a significant amount of sugar, sodium, calories, and even fat.

Cereal Choices Ratings

Rate your choice of cereals using this scale.

Outstanding: The cereal is made from whole grain and no sugar has been added.

Excellent: The cereal is made from whole grain, high in fiber, low in sugar, and low in calories.

Good: The cereal is moderate in fiber, low in sugar, and low in calories.

Okay: The cereal has a good amount of fiber but has added sugar.

Not Great: The cereal has little fiber, high sugar, high fat, or high calories — or a combination of these.

Food Tips

- When reading the ingredients list on breakfast cereals, the following ingredients should be lower than fourth on the list or even absent: sugar, brown sugar, molasses, corn syrup, organic cane juice, evaporated cane juice, high fructose corn syrup, and malt syrup.

- Choose a cereal with at least 3 grams of fiber per serving.

- To increase fiber intake, choose whole-grain cereals for breakfast or add wheat bran or wheat germ to regular cereals.

Baked Goods

Baked goods can contain significant amounts of saturated fat and are one of the biggest sources of trans fats. Hydrogenated oils tend to be used because they increase the shelf life of the foods. The saturated and trans fats become an even more serious problem with packaged baked goods shipped from a manufacturer instead of made in the store. When dairy and chocolate are used in these foods, they add significant amounts of saturated fat.

Food Tips

- When choosing baked goods, try to choose those made in the store.

- Choose the products that are made with wholegrain and have fruit added in.

- Buy only enough so that each person gets one reasonable sized serving. If there is extra left over, it will be difficult to resist eating it.

- Beware of shortening or hydrogenated oils used in the preparation of these foods.

Cakes, Muffins, and Pastries

These foods can be extremely tempting in the store. They are often all located in one large baked goods section that is difficult to miss because of the smell from the baking ovens nearby. The trouble with store-bought baked goods is that we often don't know what ingredients went into them and how much energy they provide because they lack labels.

These foods can be enjoyed but only those made with quality ingredients should be purchased. They should be eaten in the smallest amounts. A jumbo muffin can sometimes contain the full number of grain servings recommended for the entire day. Don't deprive you and your family of these types of foods, but keep the amounts reasonably small.

Cookies and Crackers

When you avoid looking at the fancy packaging on all of these foods and hone in on the ingredients list, you will discover a few things that most of these foods have in common. The first ingredient is most likely "enriched" wheat flour, which is just like pure sugar. A sugar of some sort will likely be the next main ingredient in the cookies, and then not far along will be the some form of partially hydrogenated oil, code for trans fat. In some cases, the crackers may be made with whole grains but often they are less appealing to children and the packaging is definitely less enticing. It may take you and your family some time to get used to the whole grain types of crackers, but in the end, they are the healthier option. When it comes to cookies, homemade from scratch is a better option than store-bought.

Food Tips

- Keep the portion size of these foods small because they are extremely easy to overconsume and can easily fill your child up, leaving them too full to eat more nutritious foods.

- Make sure to read the Nutrition Facts label and check serving sizes. You will likely discover that you and your child routinely eat several servings of these foods in one sitting.

Chips, Chocolates, and Candies

Everyone knows that eating too much candy, chips, and chocolate is not healthy, but repeating this warning to children doesn't make eating it any less tempting for them because of the power of advertising and the appealing taste. Instead, we have to do our best to limit the temptations causing us to purchase and consume candy, chips, and chocolate. Completely restricting these foods is not the answer because it can actually make it even more desirable. However, by never keeping any inside the house and only allowing your family to have a small amount once in a while, you will be making it easier for the family to make healthier food choices.

There are no guidelines for portions of these foods, and they should be eaten in moderation.

Food Tips

- Try to avoid the candy/chocolate/chip aisle at the grocery store. There is nothing there that you absolutely need to buy for your home.

- Always choose the smallest individually wrapped items because they discourage overeating.

- Only buy enough so that each person can have one at appropriate times.

- Beware of the candy at the checkout. When waiting in line, especially with a child, it can be very hard to resist picking something up.

Fruit Juices, Fruit Drinks, and Soda/Pop

Food Warning!

When younger children drink too many of their calories, they are likely to eat less food at meals. A line must be drawn between keeping children hydrated and giving them a constant supply of sugary drinks.

The fluids we drink on a regular basis can have an enormous effect on our daily energy intake. Regardless of whether the sugar comes from pure fruit juice, juice drinks, or soda/pop, the energy is the same. The difference between soda/pop, fruit drinks, and fruit juice is mainly in the nutrients they provide. Soda/pop provide no nutrients whatsoever and encourage tooth decay. They are simply carbonated water and sugar.

Fruit drinks may have some fruit juice content or at least some vitamins added, but like soda/pop, they are mostly water and added sugar. However, 100% fruit juice has the benefit of more vitamins, sometimes some fiber, and possibly other phytochemicals, but they are just as high in sugar as soda/pop.

As children get older, their bodies do not adjust their food intake according to the energy they get from drinks. This means that children will eat the same amount of food whether they add an extra soda/pop here and glass of juice there. There is no fiber to slow down digestion and make their stomachs feel full.

Because there is so much energy in soda/pop, fruit drinks, and fruit juices, it is easy for children to get more energy than their body needs each day. This alone is a major factor contributing to the number of children and adults who are overweight.

Q: **What is the difference between a fruit drink and a fruit juice?**

A: Fruit drinks are usually flavored water with sugar added. Occasionally, some real fruit juice will be added to these. One hundred percent fruit juice should always be chosen over fruit drinks because it only contains the juice of the fruit, possibly fiber, and no additives.

Sugar and Energy Content of Various Drinks

Beverage	Amount (ml)	Energy (Calories)	Sugar (g)	Sugar (tsp)	% Sugar
Skim/non-fat milk	240	83	13	3	5
Apple juice	240	117	29	7	12
Orange juice	240	104	25	6	10
Fruit punch	240	114	29	7	12
Cola	240	104	27	7	11
Lemon-lime soda	240	100	26	6.5	11
Gatorade	240	50	14	3.5	6
Powerade	240	65	19	5.5	8

Sports Drinks

Many children are now drinking sports drinks, which have less sugar than soda/pop or juice. These drinks are more closely matched to the amount of sugar in our blood, so our body can quickly absorb them without changing our blood sugar levels so much. Sport drinks are specifically designed to make us crave more fluid than if we were just drinking water, for example. This means that we tend to consume more of the sports drink, so even though they have less sugar than soda/pop or juice, because we drink more, we get as many or more calories. Sports drinks are unnecessary unless your child is performing endurance activities lasting longer than 1 hour.

Food Tips

- Your child is much better off getting vitamins and minerals from eating fresh fruit and vegetables than from drinking fruit juice.

- To increase fiber intake, eat whole fruits instead of drinking fruit juices.

- Soda/pop, fruit drinks and fruit juice should never be used as a thirst quencher because they may actually lead to further dehydration.

- If you are concerned that your child is not eating enough fruit and fruit juice is the only way they'll take fruit, then no more than 1 cup (250 ml) a day is recommended and it should be 100% fruit juice.

- Water should be consumed at all other times and often.

Menu Plans

With the information about fresh, whole foods and processed foods we have provided, you are ready to create menu plans that will help your children achieve a healthy weight. The menu plans we suggest are based on eating a well-balanced diet from the main food groups described in the *Food Guide Pyramid: A Guide to Daily Food Choices*, issued by the United States Department of Agriculture (USDA), or *Canada's Food Guide to Healthy Eating*, issued by Health Canada.

Three Meals and Suggested Snacks

Always aim to provide your child with three balanced meals (breakfast, lunch, and dinner) and low-caloric nutritious snacks (between breakfast and lunch and between lunch and dinner). By ensuring your children do not feel hungry throughout the day, they are less likely to overeat when food becomes available.

Building Blocks of a Meal or Snack

Try to include sources of all three macronutrients — carbohydrates, proteins, and fats — in every snack and at every meal. When all three are present, they can reduce hunger between meals. Hunger between meals can lead to cravings for high calorie snacks and can cause overeating during meals.

An example of a macronutrient balanced breakfast would be a ½ cup of yogurt (a source of carbohydrate, protein, and

Guidelines for Grocery Shopping

Before you go:

- Plan your family's meals and snacks for the week. Allow your child to be part of the decision-making process with respect to meal and snack planning. Give them specific healthy options but allow them to choose which of the options they would like. Get feedback from your child about which healthy options they like the most.

- Make a shopping list while in your kitchen and stick to it when you are at the grocery store. Knowing what you need in advance will make shopping a quicker process and will help you avoid being seduced by all the food marketing for products you don't actually need.

- Organize your shopping list in the same way as the food is found in your local grocery store.

- Eat before you go shopping so that you are not hungry and so that you do not buy impulsively.

At the grocery store:

- Remember to actually take your list to the store with you.

- Stick to your list, but make exceptions if true bargains for healthy food exist.

- Buy only the amount your family will eat before the food spoils even if it is a great bargain.

- Buy items that are divided into reasonable portion sizes. We generally eat the entire amount of any portion given to us. Buying larger sizes will only encourage over-consumption.

- Compare the cost of convenience foods with the same foods made from scratch at home such as baked goods, frozen meals, sauces. At home, you can control the fat, salt and sugar content. You also expose your child to less additives, preservatives, dyes and artificial flavors.

- Be aware that the store layout is designed to get you to buy certain items. Products placed at eye level are seen and purchased more often. End of aisle displays with a 'sale' sign may actually cost more than similar products on the shelf. These items are often less nutritious.

fat), cut up fruit (a source of carbohydrate), and a piece whole grain toast (a source of carbohydrate, protein, and fat). This menu provides sufficient amounts of all three macronutrients to keep a child satisfied, energized, and ready for school.

Mixed Macronutrient Meals and Snacks

The speed with which we can obtain nutrients from a snack or meal and the amount of time we feel satisfied depends on the types of macronutrients present.

Quick Carbs

Carbohydrates tend to be easiest for our digestive system to break down and they provide a quick source of energy.

Fat to Feel Full

Fats are broken down at a moderate speed, so they can keep us feeling full after our meal has ended and the quick carbohydrates have been processed.

Prolonged Protein

Protein takes the longest to digest and can keep us feeling full over several hours until it's time for our next meal.

CASE STUDY Ryan's Family

Cooking Again

At the bookstore Sandra searched through a number of cookbooks that focused on fast but healthy meals. It was time that the family started cooking again. No more excuses. This was too important for Ryan and the family. In her search, she happened upon a great recipe book with lots of fun, healthy snacks, especially for kid's parties. They were great! She thought that she could use some of these for Ryan's pool party. She and Ryan could go shopping for the ingredients and try out some fun, healthy snacks together. This was going to work!

The backyard was decorated with birthday balloons and colorful streamers. Although there were many traditional treats, like potato chips, candy, and birthday cake,

Ryan and his mother had made some healthy snacks as well — and they tasted great!

"This fruit salsa and cinnamon pita dip thing is amazing," commented Steve. "Yeah, and these fruit cones are so cool, I wish my mom would think of stuff like this," Josh piped in. "I'm glad you like them boys," Sandra laughed.

Ryan smiled at his mom and turned to his friends. "You guys should try the juicicles, too, we made them look like comets!" The party was a complete hit. Although Ryan was still self-conscious about his appearance, he felt good with the path his family was beginning to follow. It would only be a matter of time before they all started feeling better about themselves.

continued on page 188

Menu Building

To make eating meals and snacks more enjoyable for your children, try building a wide variety of menus by mixing and matching dishes from six food groups, adding your own family touches to them:

- Vegetables
- Fruit
- Whole grains
- Nuts, legumes and seeds
- Lean meats, poultry fish, and eggs
- Dairy and vegetable sources of calcium

Ask your children to participate in this menu building process. Each dish listed represents one serving. A summary of the recommended number of servings and portion sizes is provided at the end of this chapter and in the Healthy Weight Program chapter.

Breakfast and Snack Builder		
Vegetables	**Fruit**	**Whole Grains**
Carrot sticks	¹⁄₂ cup applesauce	30 g low-fat granola with raisins
Celery sticks	1 fruit smoothie	3-6 whole-grain crackers
Green and red peppers	1 45 g box raisins	30 g pretzels
Radish	¹⁄₂ cup fresh berries	1 small whole-wheat pita bread
Mushrooms (with or without low-fat dip or yogurt)	¹⁄₂ cup fresh fruit	80 g tortilla chips (trans fat free)
	1 cup grapes	2 blueberry pancakes
	¹⁄₂ banana	1 slice toasted bread (wheat or whole grain)
	¹⁄₂ cup strawberries	1 cup (30 g) low-sugar cereal
		2 whole-grain waffles
		1 cup raisin bran flakes or other iron-fortified cereal
		¹⁄₂ deli-sized bagel
Nuts, Legumes & Seeds	**Lean Meats, Fish, Poultry, Eggs**	**Calcium Source**
2 tbsp peanut butter	1 hard-boiled egg	1 string low-fat cheese
3 tbsp hummus	1 scrambled egg	¹⁄₂ cup low-fat cottage cheese
¹⁄₂ cup nuts or seeds	1 fried egg	1 cup (250 ml) low-fat yogurt, plain or flavored
¹⁄₂ cup (125 mL) black bean salsa	Lean cold cuts	1 cup (250 ml) low-fat milk
	Kippers	
	Smoked salmon	

Lunch Builder		
Vegetables	**Fruit**	**Whole Grains**
½ cup (50 g) sliced cucumber 10 baby carrots 1 cup (60 g) salad 1 cup (115 g) raw veggies	1 apple 1 orange 1 banana 1 pear	1 oatmeal cookie 1 slice whole-wheat bread 1 slice pizza 1 low-fat granola bar 30 g pretzels
Nuts, Legumes & Seeds	**Lean Meats, Fish, Poultry, Eggs,**	**Calcium Source**
2 tbsp peanut butter Sesame seeds or walnuts on salad	85g lean turkey 85g lean ham 85g lean beef	1 cup (250 ml) low-fat milk 1 cup (250 ml) low-fat yogurt

Dinner Builder		
Vegetables	**Fruit**	**Whole Grain**
½ cup (60 g) green beans ½ cup (75 g) steamed broccoli 1 cup tossed salad sweet potato	½ cup fresh pineapple ½ cup strawberries	1 cup (250 ml) whole wheat pasta with tomato and lean meat sauce ½ cup (100 g) steamed brown rice 2 oatmeal-raisin cookies 1 fajita wrap
Nuts, Legumes & Seeds	**Lean Meat, Fish, Poultry, Eggs,**	**Calcium Source**
½ cup almonds ½ cup walnuts	85 g roast chicken 85 g chicken breast	1 cup (250 ml) low-fat milk

Restaurant Menus

Eating out at formal and especially fast-food restaurants can present a challenge to the overweight child. Here are some tips for keeping the meal choices healthy.

General Advice
- Choose smaller portion sizes
- Limit the fried, breaded, and "crispy" dishes and replace them with more of grilled, roasted, baked, poached, broiled, and steamed dishes
- Choose lower-fat cheese on your food
- Limit your number of visits to "all you can eat" restaurants

- Choose low-fat yogurts, cottage cheese, and hard-boiled eggs for breakfast
- Mix and match menu items (if choosing a high-fat food, order a low-fat side dish)
- Ask for fresh fruits and raw vegetables or vegetable juices if vegetables are not on the menu
- Order skinless chicken menu items
- Choose salad with light or fat-free dressing
- Avoid extra unnecessary calories from bacon and cheese toppings
- Order low-fat milk or 100% juice instead of high-calorie soft drinks or fruit drinks
- Enjoy the vegetable-based soups more often than the cream-based soups.

Eating Out

Deli/Sub Shops
- Ask to add less or no mayonnaise
- Choose whole-grain breads
- Choose lower-fat meat
- Ask for lower-fat cheese

Pizza Parlors
- Choose whole wheat or multi-grain crusts when possible
- Order thin crust pizzas
- Order pizza with less cheese
- Order lower-fat cheese if available
- Choose vegetarian pizza more often
- Choose lower-fat meats such as BBQ chicken instead of pepperoni
- Using a napkin, blot the top of the pizza to soak up the extra oil
- Choose chicken breast on salad instead of deep fried wings available at some shops
- Choose a tomato-based sauce
- Be aware of the calories in garlic bread and bread sticks
- Share orders

Fast-Food Outlets
- Enjoy grilled food options more often than deep fried
- Choose various soups or salads more often than fries as a side order
- Choose baked potato instead of fries as a side
- Choose fresh fruit-based desserts more often
- Choose whole-grain buns when possible
- Reduce or leave off mayonnaise from your bun

✔ FACT

Spice of Life

Variety is essential. Changing the fruit and vegetables eaten day to day or week to week helps ensure that your child is receiving all the important nutrients needed for good health.

Servings and Portions Guidelines

Fruit and Vegetables

The goal for both children and adults should be to have at least 3 to 5 servings of vegetable and 2 to 4 servings of fruit per day. Having more than 5 servings of vegetables is just great.

Even though fruits and vegetables have different nutrient content, the number of different serving sizes is kept to a minimum to make it easy to remember. By eating a variety of fruit and vegetables, you will ensure that an adequate amount of all the nutrients are being eaten.

Legumes, Nuts, and Seeds

The goal for both children and adults should be to eat 1 or 2 servings of these foods on a daily basis. In fact, it is recommended that whole meals be based around meat alternatives, such as legumes, two or more days of the week. By eating these foods, along with whole-grain foods, it is very easy to meet daily protein needs.

Choose nuts and seeds as snacks or additions to a meal, but remember that one serving of nuts or seeds is about ¼ cup. The portion size of these foods is smaller because they have a high protein and healthy fat content and because they have high energy density. The serving sizes for the legumes, nuts, and seeds are based on the same protein and mineral content as 1 ounce (30 g) of cooked meat.

Grains

The recommendations for the number of servings of the carbohydrate foods are 5 to 11 servings per day. Ideally, all carbohydrates should be coming from whole-grain sources. It is very important to learn the amount of one serving of carbohydrates because it is easy to overconsume them. The serving sizes for the grain products are approximately equivalent to the nutrient content and calories of one thin slice of bread (between 50 and 100 Calories).

Meat, Poultry, Fish, and Eggs

An average 10-year-old child who eats a bowl of cereal with milk at breakfast, a peanut butter sandwich for lunch, and a very small amount of chicken at dinner would have all the protein needed for the day.

The recommendations for meat, poultry, fish, eggs and/or meat alternatives (such as legumes) are 2 to 3 servings per day. Children's protein needs increase as they grow into adults. One serving is 2 to 3 ounces (50 to 100 g), about the size of a deck of cards. The serving size for a younger child will be at the lower end of this range, and for an older child, it will be up at the higher end of the range.

The serving sizes for alternatives to meat are equivalent to the amount of protein in 1 ounce (30 g) of meat, poultry, or fish. One serving of alternatives provides about 7 to 10 grams of protein.

Calcium Sources

The consumption of 1 to 2 servings of low-fat dairy products per day is recommended when calcium is not being consumed from calcium-fortified beverages, such as orange juice and soy beverage, or from a calcium supplement.

The serving sizes for dairy products were chosen so that they would have approximately the same calcium content as 1 cup (250 ml) of milk, which has 300 milligrams of calcium.

The Healthy Weight Program

Eating nutritious food that does not end up being stored as fat is one key to establishing energy balance and achieving a healthy weight. Another key is increasing energy expenditure through physical activity. That is the subject of the next chapter.

CHAPTER 7
Physical Activity, Weight, and Health

While a great way of achieving a healthy weight is through good nutrition that lowers energy intake, physical activity offers another way through increasing energy expenditure. Ideally, your child will reduce excessive intake of calories and use up any extra calories in physical activity, leaving no energy to be stored as body fat, beyond the stores needed for ongoing good health.

CASE STUDY Anne's Family

Family Outing

Anne had decided it would be great for everyone to go for a hike to a beautiful waterfall and picnic spot in a park that was an hour's drive out of town. Getting everyone interested and motivated was a challenge, but she lured them with the promise of great food. Indeed, there had been wonderful smells coming from the kitchen the night before, but Anne had kept the menu top secret. As everyone got out of the car, Anne gave each of them something to carry.

The hike to the waterfall would take about an hour, and the forest smelled great and cool. They set off down the trail, Bill in front, the boys in the middle, and Anne behind. At the beginning, everyone was laughing and talking, but after half an hour and a couple of gentle hills, there was silence. Bill and Cody were huffing and puffing, and

Cody was struggling with his knapsack. They were now stopping to rest every 10 minutes, and as Anne emptied Cody's knapsack into hers and Bill's, she wondered if she had been overly optimistic.

When they finally reached the waterfall, there was little enthusiasm left, but as she spread out the blanket and laid out the feast, everyone perked up. They explored a bit after lunch and everyone paddled in the creek. The hike back to the car took longer than the hike in, and Cody and Bill slept most of the drive home. Later that evening, Bill admitted to Anne that, while he had really enjoyed the day out, he thought he was really out of shape, and that he didn't like being that way. "I used to be in great shape in high school," he explained. "We could all use more regular exercise," she agreed, and she started to think of a plan.

continued on page 190

The Value of Physical Activity

All health professionals and research scientists agree that physical activity is essential for maintaining overall good health. The health benefits of regular physical activity and exercise are tremendous.

Better Quality of Life

Physical activity contributes to a better quality of life. It can decrease the likelihood of sickness and lead to a longer and healthier life. It leads to increased feelings of well-being, with decreased anxiety, worries, and depression. We may feel more relaxed and more confident in our abilities. We have improved self-esteem. Physical activities may take us into social settings where we have opportunities to strengthen friendships, meet new people, and improve our social support circle.

Better Performance

A physically active body is one that performs well. The heart, lungs, and the muscles of the body become stronger and more efficient. Physical activity may improve flexibility, coordination, and balance, which improve posture. Being physically fit improves not only our abilities to perform physical activities required by school or work, but also our performance in recreation and sports.

Better Health

Physical activity is important for the strength of our bones and muscles. We burn off calories during exercise, so it also important for helping us to keep a healthy weight. It reduces both total body fat and central body fat. When we are physically active, we are transforming the energy from the foods we eat and from our store of energy in body fat into the energy of movement. Energy is required to fuel these movements: the harder or more vigorous the movement, the more energy that is required and the more energy that is expended. Physical activity and decreasing our body fatness helps to control high blood cholesterol, high blood pressure, and diabetes. In children, physical activity is important for healthy growth and development.

 FACT

School Exercises

The Canadian Association for Health, Physical Education, Recreation, and Dance advocates that, during school hours, all Canadian children participate in at least 30 minutes of physical education every day from kindergarten through Grade 12. The Canadian Medical Association passed a resolution in 1998 calling for 30 minutes per day of compulsory physical education for every child. However, many schools don't provide this.

Physical Activity Settings

Physical activity is required in many settings in our day-to-day lives. It is not limited to periods of structured exercise.

Body System

The body is physically active even when it is completely still or at rest or asleep, keeping the lungs breathing and the heart pumping, as well as maintaining posture. The energy needed for these basic body functions is called the basal metabolic rate (BMR). Children and adolescents also grow, another form of physical activity.

Home

As part of our normal routine of living in the home, we are physically active, walking up the stairs, washing dishes, vacuuming, sweeping, taking out the garbage, and more. We rarely think of these activities as structured exercise, we just do them. However, North American children are doing fewer daily living activities these days. There is a relationship between the decrease in these types of activities and the increase in overweight for children.

Work and School

Different jobs will require different levels of physical activity, ranging from heavy construction work, for example, to relatively sedentary office work. Children may walk to class or the bus stop, walk between classes, and participate in physical education classes. There is also a decrease in the amount of physical activity children experience in school settings with the increase in bus services and the decrease in time allotted to physical education.

Organized Sports

At school or in the community, children may participate in organized sports activities, whether they be team-based, one-on-one, or solo sports. The level of activity and types of movement or skills are specific to the demands of the sport. Often, there is an element of competition. Sports can be an effective way for children to become more physically active.

Fitness Exercise

With exercise, the goal is fitness. Fitness exercise is planned, structured, and repetitive. Physical fitness usually refers to our physical ability to perform movements. Physical fitness also includes our attitude towards physical activity, specifically, whether we ourselves believe that we have the ability to do achieve a fitness goal and whether we believe fitness is important. Leading your children to believe in their ability to reach fitness goals is an important role you can play.

Play
This is any activity performed for the intent of having fun. There are no specific fitness goals or structured activities, although a lot of energy may be used in play. This is the best type of activity for younger children because it is focused first on having fun. By encouraging your children to play, you are helping them to achieve a healthy weight and maintain good health.

Types of Physical Activity

Physical activities can be categorized into several roles for achieving better quality of life, better health, including healthy weight, and better performance.

1. Daily Living Activities
2. Endurance Activities
3. Strength Activities
4. Flexibility Activities

All four types of physical activity have one thing in common: they involve contracting or squeezing the muscles to hold up or to move the body. Any time the muscles are squeezing, this is physical activity.

Daily Living Activities
These are the activities we perform as we go about our daily routines. Because these activities are rarely thought of as exercise, they can be one easy way to add activity to your child's day with little effort. These usual activities are actually just as important as regular exercise for maintaining a healthy weight.

Endurance Activities
Endurance or aerobic activities involve continuous muscle movement over a long period of time, requiring a constant supply of energy and oxygen. These activities get the heart and lungs working harder and faster, often causing us to sweat.

Moderate endurance activities increase the heart rate and increase breathing, but generally not to a degree where talking becomes difficult. Some examples of moderate activities include walking quickly, riding a bike, skating, and playing outdoors. Vigorous activities get things moving even faster,

 FACT

Enduring Benefits
Many of the greatest benefits of regular physical activity actually come from endurance activities. These aerobic activities are especially important for developing and maintaining a strong healthy heart and lungs. They are also important for helping your child achieve and keep a healthy body weight.

causing the heart to pound and a feeling of shortness of breath. We also sweat more and often can't carry on a conversation. Running sports, such as track and field, soccer, and basketball, are examples of vigorous activities.

Strength Activities

Strength activities involve forceful or powerful movements lasting only a short time. The movements are performed against resistance or opposition. They may involve moving one's own body weight or moving extra weight against gravity. Weight lifting and bodybuilding are strength building activities, as are chin-ups or sit-ups, climbing hills or stairs, jumping on a trampoline, gymnastics, dance, and martial arts.

These activities may have endurance parts to them as well. For example, although dance can have a lot of jumps or holding postures that take strength, there is also a lot of moving around. Some of the endurance activities may have strength parts as well. For example, in basketball, there is a lot of running but also jumping.

Extra Value of Strength Activities

Besides lowering body fat, strength activities have several other health benefits:

- Strength activities help your child develop strong muscles and bones. Having strong muscles can improve your child's performance in sport or play.

- Strength activities can also help to prevent disease and injuries, such as bone fractures.

- Before puberty, strength activities do not cause the muscles to get larger like a body builder, but the muscles do get much stronger and toned. Having a strong body can make children feel better about their body and themselves, giving them a feeling of confidence about participating in physical activities and sports.

- Strength activities help connections form between the brain and the muscles to coordinate muscle movement. These connections need to form in childhood because as children grow into adults, the connections are much harder to form.

- Having strong, toned muscles is also important for maintaining healthy weight because each pound of lean muscle burns an additional 30 to 50 Calories per day, even if it is not being used.

- Each pound of muscle also takes up 30% less space than a pound of fat.

Flexibility Activities

Flexibility activities involve stretching the ligaments and tendons that connect the muscles to the bones or one bone to another, allowing us to bend, reach, and stretch. Flexibility is important in keeping the body able to move through a full range of movements. Some examples of activities that focus on improving flexibility include gymnastics and dance. Specifically, stretching exercises are used to warm up for or cool down from other types of activities. Flexibility activities are especially important after strength or endurance activities to prevent muscle soreness and stiffness.

Inflexible joints may reduce your child's ability to perform to their best potential in activities. Inflexible joints are also more prone to injury. Flexibility activities also have a calming effect on the muscles and on the mind and can help your child relax.

Q: How does physical activity relate to bone development?

A: When bones develop during childhood, they become thicker and stronger. Children who are physically active and get lots of calcium from their nutrition have the thickest and strongest bones by the end of puberty. After puberty, the bones stop growing and actually start to slowly lose some of their weight throughout adulthood. If this happens at a fast rate, osteoporosis or brittle bones develop, making the bones easier to break. Being physically active as a child means that they start out with stronger bones and are less likely to develop osteoporosis as they become older adults.

Energy and Activity

We need to take in a certain amount of calories to meet basic energy needs, with the remaining calories going toward fueling physical activity. The body needs a certain amount of energy to maintain basal metabolic rate (BMR) even when it is still, at rest, or asleep, in order to keep the lungs breathing and the heart pumping and to maintain posture. Even when the body is standing or sitting still, the muscles are flexing in order to give support and balance. Children and adolescents also need energy for growth and development. These are the body's minimum needs for energy, something over which we have little control.

However, we do control the amount of daily living, endurance, strength, and flexibility activity we get. By increasing our physical activity, we use more energy, including the energy stored mainly as body fat. Using this stored energy and reducing body fat is not as easy as it sounds. It is a lot easier for us to take in extra calories than it is to burn them off with physical activity. By nature, people find it easy to eat but not so easy to get moving. We can eat a candy bar in about 2 minutes, but we may need to exercise for 30 minutes to use up the energy from that candy bar. To use up this energy takes a lot of movement. Any energy left over is stored as fat.

Energy Stores

Food can be thought of as fuel for our body, derived from the breakdown of chemical bonds of all three macronutrients (carbohydrates, fats, and proteins). Carbohydrates provide immediate energy. Fat stores offer a secondary energy source. Protein is generally only used for fuel in periods of fasting or starvation, when carbohydrate and fat macronutrients are not available. When this happens, the body resorts to breaking down its own muscle to survive. This is called catabolism.

Q: **Can diets be harmful for children?**

A: When most people hear the word diet, they think of restricting the amount of food eaten. When food (fuel) is restricted, the body slows down its functions in order to conserve energy. Some of the body's essential functions cannot be slowed down very much, such as generating heat to keep the body warm. If the food we eat does not provide us with enough energy to fuel the body's vital functions, our body uses the energy stored in our fat but it also breaks down our muscle to provide energy. This is harmful in children because their bodies should be growing and their muscles should be increasing in size.

Glucose and Glycogen

All carbohydrates get broken down into simple sugars, such as glucose, which is then used for energy in the body. When there is more glucose in the body than it needs, the extra glucose can be stored in the muscles as a more complex chemical called glycogen. The liver also stores glucose as glycogen. Glycogen can be quickly broken down into an immediate supply of glucose, which can then be used instantly to provide energy to working muscles.

The glycogen stores are not large and they cannot get bigger the way our fat stores can. Imagine that glycogen stores are like a paper bag, whereas fat stores are more like a balloon. Also, imagine that glycogen is for short-term storage, like a refrigerator, compared to long-term storage of fat, more like a freezer. Once the glycogen stores are full in the muscle and the liver, which can happen after a meal with lots of carbohydrates, the extra glucose then gets stored as fat for longer-term energy storage.

Fat

The process of breaking down the stored fat to provide the muscles with energy is slow. It also requires a lot of oxygen, which we get from the air we breathe. In contrast, glycogen can be instantly broken down to glucose, which then directly provides energy to the muscles, even when oxygen levels are lower.

Energy Systems

Anaerobic System

The anaerobic system, also known as the glycogen-lactic acid system, relies on breaking down stored muscle glycogen to supply energy to the muscles. This system for providing energy is called anaerobic because it does not need oxygen. This system is ready to work as soon as it is needed, but it can only provide continuous energy for about 90 seconds before it needs to recover.

As a result of breaking down glycogen and glucose, the anaerobic system creates waste products, such as carbon dioxide and lactic acid. Carbon dioxide is a gas that is simply removed from our body as we breathe. However, lactic acid can build up in the muscle and interfere with the anaerobic system's ability to continue to supply energy. This limits the amount of time that the anaerobic system is useful. Lactic acid can also interfere with muscle action and cause the soreness in our muscles we sometimes feel during or after exercise. Higher levels of lactic acid in the blood can keep us breathing at a slightly faster than normal rate for minutes to hours after the physical activity is stopped. Our liver will remove lactic acid from our blood. The body may continue to need more energy for this process even after the physical activity is finished.

Glycogen Versus Fat

Glycogen: Short-term storage of glucose. Quickly provides energy for muscle work. Doesn't need a lot of oxygen.

Fat: Long-term storage of energy. Slowly provides energy for muscle work. Needs a good supply of oxygen.

✔ **FACT**

On Your Mark, Get Set, Go …
The anaerobic system is especially useful during strength and more vigorous or faster endurance activities, such as weight training (resistance training), at the start of a running race, and during soccer when a sprint for the ball is needed.

Aerobic System

The anaerobic system can become exhausted, at which point the aerobic system must help out and provide energy if physical activity is to continue. Unlike the anaerobic system, oxygen is needed at the outset. The aerobic system involves more chemical reactions than the anaerobic system and provides energy at a slower rate.

When the need for energy is low to moderate, the aerobic system mainly breaks down fat. Fats may either come from a recently eaten meal or from our fat stores. As the need for energy increases, the aerobic system will start using more short-term energy supplies, such as glucose or glycogen.

Unlike the anaerobic system, this system can continue to supply energy as long as oxygen and fuel are available. This system is always in use, whether we are sleeping, sitting, walking, or running, and provides energy for endurance activities, such as long-distance running, biking, rowing, and cross-country skiing.

Systems Interactions

The aerobic system is in use at all times during all activities. It becomes especially important for supplying energy when performing endurance physical activities. This is because the anaerobic system can only be used for a very short period of time before it becomes exhausted and not as useful for supplying energy. If the endurance activity is vigorous and needs a lot of energy, then the aerobic system must work faster. In this situation, the aerobic system will rely more on glycogen and glucose rather than fat for fuel, and the anaerobic system will also be working. If the endurance activity is less vigorous, then only the aerobic system is needed and fat will be used for fuel.

Regular physical activity will help your child to improve all of these functions and will help the aerobic system to work better. If the aerobic system is working well, your child will be able to perform physical activity for a longer period of time. They will also feel less uncomfortable and out of breath while they are exercising.

✔ **FACT**

Healthy Heart
Regular physical activity for long enough periods of time will improve the health and fitness of the heart and lungs, and will also help to keep a healthy body weight by burning off extra calories.

Anaerobic System Assistance

There are three circumstances when the anaerobic system is needed to help the aerobic system to supply muscles with energy:

1. When just starting endurance physical activity

As the body begins performing an endurance physical activity, the muscles start needing more energy. At the start of the activity, the heart and lungs are still in a resting state. It may take a while for the heart to pump faster and stronger and the lungs to breathe faster and deeper in order to give the muscles the greater amounts of oxygen and nutrients that are required. Since there is not yet enough oxygen available for the aerobic system, the anaerobic system (which does not need oxygen) provides the energy at the start.

2. When the aerobic system cannot supply sufficient energy

The aerobic system is a slower system than the anaerobic system. When the muscles need to work extra hard for a short period of time, such as when sprinting, they have bigger energy needs. These needs can occur so quickly that the aerobic system does not have enough time to supply the necessary amount of energy. When this happens, the anaerobic system helps out.

3. When the need for oxygen is greater than the amount of oxygen that is available

This is especially important for children who are inactive and overweight. During any type of physical activity, whenever the amount of oxygen available is not enough to meet the needs of the aerobic system, the anaerobic system must help out in order to provide enough energy to continue the activity. However, the anaerobic system can only be used for a short period of time, after which the activity may become impossible to continue because energy is not available. This may occur for unfit individuals who perform endurance physical activity. This happens for several reasons:

- The lungs are not large and healthy enough to quickly supply a large amount of oxygen.

- The red blood cells are weak and cannot carry enough oxygen through the bloodstream to the muscles to fill the greater need in the muscles.

- The heart may be unfit and not be able to pump the blood to the muscles quickly enough to fill the need for oxygen and nutrients.

- The muscles themselves may be underdeveloped and unable to accept the greater amounts of blood with oxygen and nutrients.

- The aerobic system may be underdeveloped and inefficient, unable to supply the energy needed.

CASE STUDY Ryan's Family

Plan for Action

Sandra and her husband, Greg, now realized the importance of making changes to lead a healthier lifestyle, not only for Ryan's sake, but for everyone in the family. While he had tried to ignore it, deep down Greg knew that his weight and lifestyle would catch up to him sooner or later.

They discussed reducing many of the convenience dinners, including weekly visits to fast-food outlets and ordering in pizza.

Looking at the pantry, they were amazed at how much junk they left out for the kids to just grab and go. They also discussed exercise. They agreed that for nights when Dave did not have soccer that they would try to have a family bike ride. They would also get more use from the pool in the backyard, buying some pool toys and trying some new pool games. They were going to tackle this together.

Energy Balance

Each of the four categories of physical activity (daily living, endurance, strength, and flexibility) plays a special role for getting and keeping a healthy body weight. The importance of all of these types of activities in healthy weight management is to get a good balance between our energy intake, or the amount of fuel or calories we eat, and our energy expenditure, or the amount of energy we actually use. The balance on the scale will determine whether or not there is excess fuel that will be stored as fat.

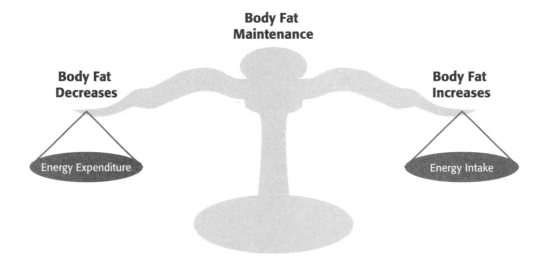

If your child is currently getting more energy from the foods they are eating (energy intake) than what they are using up (energy expenditure), the excess energy will be stored as body fat. If your child is not active enough throughout the day, the energy expenditure will be lower than what is healthy and the scale will tip even further toward increasing body fat. The importance of physical activity is that it helps tip the scale back toward weight maintenance and an ideal energy balance.

When a healthy amount of physical activity is balanced with a healthy energy intake, your child will no longer have extra energy to store as body fat. In addition, as children grow and develop, their weight will become better balanced for their height. Many parents may not be concerned about their child's weight because they believe that they will just "grow into it." The problem is that unless the energy balance is corrected, extra fat will continue to be stored and soon height growth will run out. For these children, it may be necessary to decrease energy intake and increase physical activity to help tip the scale toward fat loss.

While cutting out excess calories is the most efficient way to tip the energy balance, increasing daily activity (especially if originally we are inactive) considerably increases the total amount of calories the body uses up each day. When this is combined with eating more reasonable amounts of healthy foods, the body will use up all the calories from the food we eat and even some of the excess fat stores.

Q: Will increasing my children's physical activity make them hungrier and eat more?

A: You might think that if your daughter or son does more physical activity and uses up more energy that they will feel hungry and eat more than usual. It is true that they will be using up more energy and that they may in fact want to eat more. However, research shows that a small to moderate increase in exercise does not lead to increased food intake. Also, if the increased foods they eat are healthy, they are less likely to take in more energy than what they are using up.

Energy Efficiency

One of the problems we face when trying to restore energy balance through physical activity is that the body is incredibly energy efficient.

- An average sized car may go 6 to 12 kilometers for each liter or 16 to 24 miles for each gallon of gasoline it uses, while the amount of calories in just 1 liter or quart of gasoline would allow a person to walk 120 kilometers or 80 miles.

- About 100 calories is enough energy to allow the average 10-year-old child to walk briskly for an hour at a pace of 3 miles per hour or 5 kilometers per hour.

- Eating a small order of fast-food French fries provides 10 grams of fat ($\frac{1}{6}$ of the recommended daily fat intake) and 210 Calories. To use up the energy from the fries, a child would need to walk briskly for 2 hours! If a large-sized order of fries is eaten, this means 4 hours of walking. The body can go a long way on a few calories.

- Two small cookies with about 100 Calories can allow a child to walk 5 kilometers or 3 miles.

Just by eating a few small cookies here and an order of fries there, the extra calories can quickly add up.

CASE STUDY Anne's Family

Setting Some Goals

Anne held the brochure up for everyone to see. "I am going to enter this 5-K race coming up in 3 months, but I'm going to need some help from all of you for me to get in shape so that I can do it," she said. They were skeptical. She was in the best shape of all of them.

Bill took her hint and said, "Count me in. I could jog with you sometimes. Maybe I will try to run the race with you. What about you boys?" Mark was excited. "I bet I could beat you Dad." Cody didn't know what to think. "It would be great if everyone in the family did the race, but we would all have to work together and help each other out," Anne explained.

They thought about how they would all get in shape. They would start slowly and gradually build up their speed and distance.

Anne suggested that Cody could be her training coach, and that Mark could coach Bill. The boys loved that idea, and started thinking of what they would do each day for the next week. "Why wait for next week. We can start right now," Bill volunteered. "We can start by agreeing that there will only be 1 hour of television each day," suggested Mark. "Except for Saturday mornings," added Cody.

"That's a great goal!" exclaimed Anne. "We could wear matching T-shirts for the race, maybe even with our own design," said Mark. For the next half hour they wrote out a training plan. They would be well-prepared for race day, and everyone was confident that they could finish, in style.

continued on page 212

Measuring METs

The amount of activity the body can do for each calorie of food energy depends on the type of physical activity and how long the activity is carried out. There are two common ways of describing the energy needs for doing various physical activities.

Calories

The number of calories of energy used is one way. For example, if an average child walks briskly for an hour, 100 Calories of energy will be used. If the same child runs for the same amount of time, they will use 300 Calories of energy. However, few children are perfectly average, and the amount of energy needed to do the same type and amount of activity may not be the same. This depends on the age and size of the child and their level of physical fitness. It takes more energy to move extra weight, so an overweight child may need or use more energy than a lean child to do the same amount of physical activity.

MET (Metabolic Equivalent)

We can also use another measure of energy needs called the MET, which can be more useful since it does not differ as much depending on the individual. The energy of one MET is about the amount of energy that is used by the body when it

MET Levels of Various Activities	
Activity	**METs**
Sleeping	1
Lying awake	1.2
Sitting quietly	1.2
Standing quietly	1.4
Walking slowly	2.8
Walking at normal pace	3.2
Walking uphill fast	7.5
Moderate recreation and sports (dancing, swimming, tennis)	3 to 6
Vigorous recreation and sports (soccer, jogging, running, rowing)	more than 6

Modified from: www.cps.ca/english/statements/HAL/HAL02-01.htm

is just sitting still or at rest. To walk briskly, the body would need about three times this amount of resting energy, or 3 METs. We can use METs to rate the energy needed for any type of physical activity. The greater the number of METs, the more energy the physical activity needs and uses. The more energy used for the activity, the more calories your child will use up doing it.

Healthy Weight METs

Measuring METS

The amount of energy used up doing each activity will depend on the number of METs needed for the activity and the amount of time spent doing the activity. Starting with the body's energy needs at rest, or 1 MET, we can change this to the speed at which calories are used. Although not everyone has the same energy needs at rest, we can use METs to give us a good estimation about our own individual speed of energy expenditure while doing various activities.

For an example, we will suppose that a particular person uses energy at a speed of 1 Calorie every minute at rest — or at 1 MET. Walking takes 3 METs, whereas jogging takes 6 METs. Since walking uses 3 METs and each MET, for this particular person, equals 1 Calorie used per minute, walking uses 3 Calories every minute. Also, since jogging takes 6 METs, jogging would use 6 Calories every minute. Jogging takes twice as many METs as walking for the same amount of time.

The greater the number of METs an activity needs, the harder it is to do the activity. Thus, jogging takes twice the amount of effort as walking. It also takes the body half the time to use up the same amount of energy during jogging than during walking. If we need to use up some extra calories, we can either go for a short jog or a long walk.

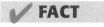

FACT

METs + Time
METs and time gives us energy expenditure. This is a very important idea to understand as we discuss the role of the four main types of physical activity for getting and keeping a healthy body weight.

Q: **How much water should my child be drinking before, during, and after physical activity?**

A: During continuous activity lasting longer than 30 minutes, fluid should be replaced at a rate of 100 ml to 150 ml every 15 to 30 minutes, even if your child doesn't feel thirsty.

Daily Activity METs

Doing everyday activities are important for getting and keeping a healthy weight. The body uses a considerable amount of energy while doing routine things. The amount of time spent doing an activity is a large part of the amount of energy used. For example, you may think that having your child jog for a half hour is better exercise than walking to school, playing on the playground, helping to clear the dinner table and washing up, or playing a board game before bed, but this is not necessarily true.

There are, in fact, advantages to endurance activities with high METs, like jogging or running, but the energy used over a day doing routine things can add up. If one MET is equal to using energy at a speed of 1 Calorie every minute, then 30 minutes of jogging (at 6 METs) will use up about 180 Calories.

✔ FACT • Sedentary Switch

Encouraging your child to increase daily living activities that seem easy and need a smaller number of METs, but are done for longer periods of time, is a valuable way to increase the amount of energy the body uses up. Activities that don't seem difficult (such as walking) and many activities that are fun (such as playing tag) use up an important amount of energy. Any physical activity will use up more energy than watching television. Switch off the television and switch sedentary recreation (watching television, playing computer or video games, surfing the Internet, or just sitting around) with any type of physical activity, especially fun and interesting activities.

The activities of daily living also use up an important amount of energy. Walking to school, walking around at school during lunch and recess, and then walking home could add up to 1 or 2 hours of activity alone. At 3 METs for walking, that could mean up to about 400 Calories used, about two times more calories used than with the half hour of jogging or running. If we add playing on the playground (5 METs) for 30 minutes, another 150 Calories are used. Clearing the dinner table and washing up (2.5 METs) done for even 15 minutes will use up another 40 Calories. Playing a board game (1.5 METs) for a half hour before bed will use up 45 Calories.

If we add all that up, we have about 635 Calories used in daily living activities. If we take away the play after school and replace it with an hour of television watching (1 MET), the total amount of calories used drops to 500 Calories. If we also take away an hour of walking to and from school, the total energy used drops to about 350 Calories. Clearly, the activities of daily living are a very important part of the body's total daily energy expenditure.

Moderate and Vigorous Endurance Activity METs

Endurance, strength, and flexibility activities have their own role to play in helping your child get and keep a healthy weight. The effort needed to do these various activities can be graded as either moderate or vigorous. Physical activities that are considered moderate in effort usually have MET levels from 3 to 6. Vigorous activities have MET levels greater than 6. The activities of daily living often have MET levels of around 3 or less.

By participating in regular physical activity, both of moderate and vigorous effort, your child will improve their total fitness and gain all the health benefits of physical activity. Regular physical activity will also help your child to lose extra body fat. Research has shown that regular physical activity is the best way to get and keep a healthy weight. Regular physical activity can also help control your child's feelings of hunger and their food intake.

Q: **How much moderate and vigorous physical activity should my child get each day?**

A: The recommendations for the amount of daily physical activity for children are at least 60 minutes of moderate activity and 30 minutes of vigorous activity. The goal is to replace the inactive time (screen time: television, video games, and computer) with moderate and vigorous activity, while keeping the activities of daily living the same or increasing them as well. When your child meets these recommendations, they will use up a larger amount of energy and they will be making progress toward getting and keeping a healthy body weight. The recommendations are also easier to follow than trying to calculate the exact energy expenditure of each activity using METs and calories.

Strength Activity METS

Doing strength activities can use lots of energy. Most strength activities have high MET levels. Because some of the strength activities with high METs are very difficult, they cannot be done for as long as other types of activities. For this reason, your child may not wish to spend a lot of time or use a lot energy in strength activities.

However, there are more benefits to strength activities than just using up calories. Strength activities are important to help your child develop stronger and more toned muscle. The stronger and more toned the muscles, the more energy is needed to keep them that way. Lean muscle also gives your child's body a more fit appearance, which can help build confidence and self-esteem. Doing strength activities is a better choice than watching television, but it is possible to do some strength activities and watch television at the same time. One specific type of strength activity is resistance training, such as working against a weight. Regular resistance training can be a good part of the activity program for your child to help them become stronger and more fit.

Flexibility Activity METs

Flexibility activities, such as gymnastics and dance, have high MET levels and can also be considered endurance activities. Activities that increase flexibility are important for preventing injuries, which will keep your child participating and performing well whatever the activity.

Not all children want to participate in activities that naturally increase flexibility, so it may be important for your child to put some flexibility exercises into daily activity routines. Flexibility activities, such as stretching exercises, should be done after endurance and strength activities. Stretching after these activities can prevent muscle soreness and stiffness and allow a faster recovery. Learning proper stretching exercise methods and developing a habit of stretching will help make sure that your child stays flexible throughout their lifetime.

✔ **FACT**

Setting Targets
There is no reason to start calculating the calories and METs for every activity your child will be doing. Setting targets or goals for the amount of time spent doing moderate and vigorous activities each day is a simpler method and just as successful.

Q: What is cross-training?

A: Cross-training means participating in all categories of physical activity and a variety from each category — moderate and vigorous endurance, strength, and flexibility. Children need to develop all of their muscles, not just the ones for a specific activity.

Cross-training also develops coordination. When your child moves their body, their brain learns these movement patterns. For example, as your child learned to walk, a motor program was developed in their brain. You can think of this as the walking program. It instructs all the muscles when to move, how much force to apply, and so on. With cross-training, your child will develop all sorts of motor programs that can all be used together when performing other new activities. There is a window of opportunity during childhood when it is easiest to develop the motor programs, but as your child grows toward adulthood, it becomes much more difficult.

Cross-training also makes participating in physical activity more fun and enjoyable and less boring so your child is much more likely to be active.

Full-Body Strength-Training and Stretching Program

We have provided a 12-stage workout that will ensure that your children are exercising the major muscle groups in the body. Each strength exercise is paired with a flexibility exercise that stretches the muscles they have worked. The strength exercises are all done first, followed by all the paired stretching exercises. The stretching exercises are presented in the order in which they should be done.

Supervision

Be sure to supervise your children as they perform the strength-training activities in the workout. By being present, you can provide motivation and ensure that they are using safe technique.

Focus on teaching them the proper technique for all exercises, making safety and injury avoidance the number one priority. Some of the exercises can be made more challenging by changing technique or by applying more resistance or weight. This should only be done once technique is perfect and it should be done gradually. Remember, no matter how big or strong your children appear, their bodies are still immature.

Warm-Up

Before having your child perform any strength or flexibility activities, get the blood flowing to their muscles and warm them. Without a warm-up, muscles will not work as well and they may even become injured.

- Intensity: The warm-up should not be difficult. Your child should be able to carry on a conversation easily during the entire warm up.
- Duration: 3 to 5 minutes is all that is needed to warm up and the best activities are ones that use the whole body.
- Types of warm-up activities:
  - Brisk walking or light jogging on the spot, around the house, or outside. The feet should not be hitting the ground hard.
  - Big arm movements are important to warm up the arms.
  - Light skipping.
  - Bicycling or pedaling on a stationary bike.

Strength (Resistance) Training Principles

(Based on the American College of Sports Medicine guidelines for children and resistance training.)

- Proper breathing: Throughout each exercise, ensure that your children are not holding their breath. One way to help teach them this is to have them count out the number of the rep they are completing.
- Proper speed: Ensure that your children perform each exercise in a manner in which the speed is controlled. Fast and jerky movements are less effective and more risky. As a general rule, have your child count 2 to 3 seconds for the first half of each repetition and 2 to 3 seconds for the second half of each repetition.
- Rest between strength exercises: Initially, children may need rest to catch their breath between each exercise. This is normal. As they become more fit, they should aim to move from exercise to exercise without stopping to rest.
- Recovery: Every time a workout routine is completed, you should allow 2 or 3 days to pass before repeating it. Your child should only complete the routine for a maximum of two times per week to allow recovery and prevent boredom with the routine. On other days during the week, help your child become involved with other forms of physical activity.
- Intensity: Some exercises can be done with only your child's own body weight as resistance. Others may require small weights or dumbbells.

✔ **FACT**

Don't Overdo It!

If adding resistance to strength exercises, your child should still be able to perform 8 reps keeping perfect form. Otherwise, injury can result. Stretching should never hurt. Perform the stretching exercises only to the point where a slight tension is felt in the muscle.

- Goals: The final goal is for your child to be able to perform one exercise for 8 to 12 repetitions and to build up to performing a set of all 12 exercises. Initially, young people may not be able to complete 8 repetitions. Reassure them that with practice more repetitions can be completed.
- Good form: Make sure your child keeps good form or there is no point to increasing the number of repetitions.
- Stretching: After completing strength exercises, all muscle groups worked should be stretched. Always try to relax the muscles being stretched completely.

Rep

One complete exercise movement is a rep (repetition). For example, one rep of an arm curl (bicep curl) would be bringing the fist (or weight) from the bottom position to the top position and lowering it again in a controlled manner.

Set

One set is the completion of a specific number (or repetitions) of an exercise. For example, a set of bicep curls could be 12 reps.

12-Stage Full-Body Strength and Stretching Program				
Combo	Strength Exercise	Muscle Group	Stretching Exercise	Time
1	Squats	Front of legs (quadriceps)	Quadricep Stretches	2 min
2	Lunges	Back of legs (hamstrings)	Hamstring Stretches	2 min
3	Calf Raises	Lower legs (calves)	Calf Stretches	2 min
4	Leg Raises	Outer thighs (leg abductors)	Leg Stretches	2 min
5	Pelvic Raises	Gluteals (buttocks)	Buttocks Stretches	2 min
6	Bent-over Rows	Upper back	Upper Back Stretches	2 min
7	Wall Push-ups	Pectorals (chest muscles)	Chest stretches	2 min
8	Lateral Arm Raises	Shoulders (deltoid)	Shoulder Stretches	2 min
9	Biceps Curls	Biceps (front of arms)	Biceps Stretches	2 min
10	Tricep Dip	Triceps (back of arms)	Triceps Stretches	2 min
11	Back Extensions	Humbar (lower back muscles)	Lower Back Stretches	2 min
12	Stomach Crunches	Stomach (abdominal muscles)	Abdominal Stretches	2 min
				24 min

FULL-BODY STRENGTH-TRAINING AND STRETCHING COMBINATION EXERCISES

Combo 1: Quadriceps, Hamstrings, Gluteals (Upper Legs)
Squats

- Stand straight with your stomach muscles tight and your feet shoulder width apart. Hold your hands together in front of you for balance. This is your starting position.
- Slowly sit back as if you were going to sit in a chair, pressing through the heels and lowering over 4 seconds. Make sure your knees do not move forward past your toes, you're looking straight ahead and your back is straight. Imagine sticking your buttocks far back behind you. From the seated position, with knees bent at no less than a 90-degree angle, press into the floor through your heals and come back to the starting position.
- Repeat this movement 8 to 12 times.
- Correcting form: Watch that the knees do not move forward past the toes. Make sure the upper body is almost vertical through the whole movement and the weight is in the heels.

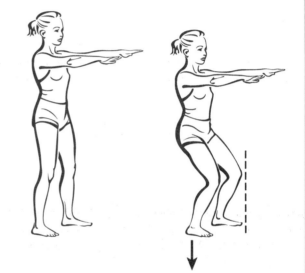

Quadricep Stretches

- Using a wall for support and balance, stand on your right leg. Keeping the knee slightly bent, tuck your hips forward. Flex your left knee and reach back with your left hand to grab your left ankle. Move your right knee back away from you while resisting with your left hand. Feel the stretch and hold for 15–30 seconds.
- Standing on your left leg, flex your right knee and reach back with your right hand to grab your right ankle. Move your left knee back away from you while resisting with your right hand. Feel the stretch and hold for 15–30 seconds.
- Repeat this stretch twice for each leg.
- Correcting form: Keep the upper body straight and the bent knee in line beside the knee of the straight leg. Keep the upper body straight over the hips. Do not arch the back or lean forward, backward, or to one side.

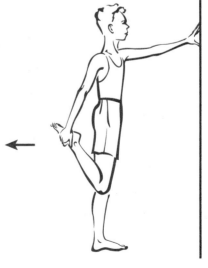

Combo 2: Hamstrings, Quadriceps, Gluteals (Upper Legs)

Lunges

* Stand with your feet slightly apart and grasp the back of a sturdy chair. Stand far enough back from the chair so that your arms are fully extended but your upper body is straight. This is your starting position.
* Step forward with your right foot so that your toe is just in front of the chair. Keep your upper body and head in a straight vertical line during the entire movement.
* Put your weight in your right heel as you bend your right knee and slowly lower yourself until your left knee just touches the floor. Be sure that your right knee does not move forward past your right toes. Now, pushing through your right heel, raise your body up slowly and step back to the starting position over 2 to 4 seconds.
* Repeat these movements 8 to 12 times with your right leg and then with your left leg.
* Correcting form: Watch that the front knee does not move forward past the front toes. The hips, upper body and head should all be in a vertical line.

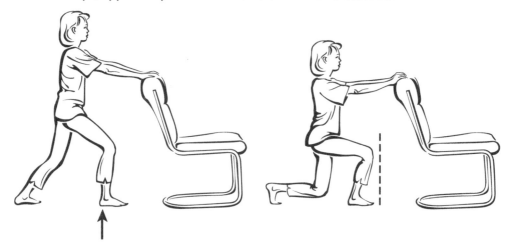

Hamstring Stretches

* Lie on your back with knees bent and feet flat on the floor. Bring one knee toward your chest and extend this leg, pressing the sole of the foot toward the ceiling.
* The knee joint should not be locked. With the leg straight in the air, try to gently bring the leg closer to your chest until you feel a stretch.
* Repeat twice for each leg.

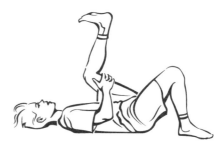

Combo 3: Calves (Lower Legs)

Calf Raises

- Stand on a step and grasp a railing or the wall for support. Your body should be straight and tall and your knees should never be locked straight. Move your feet back so that your heels are hanging over the edge of the step. Allow your heels to drop just below the level of the step. This is your starting position.
- From here, slowly raise up on the balls of your feet (the bottom of your feet that comes before your toes) for 4 seconds so that you are as high as possible. You should be able to feel the contraction in your calves.
- Lower back down to the starting position over 4 seconds.
- Repeat this movement 8 to 12 times.
- Correcting form: The movement is slow and never bouncy or jerky. Holding a railing is only for balance and should not be helping in the movement. Make sure to rise high enough on the balls of the feet to create the stretch. Knees should be slightly bent through the entire movement.

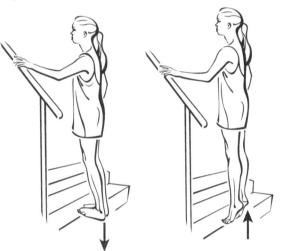

Calf Stretches

- Stand at arm's length in front of a wall, placing your hands on the wall at the level of your chest, shoulder width apart.
- Step with the ball of your right foot back and bend your front leg as you slowly lower your right heel down to the floor, feeling a stretch in the lower leg. Your back leg should be straight but your knee should not be locked. Hold this stretch for 15 to 30 seconds.
- Repeat on the other side.

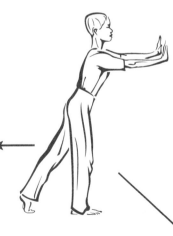

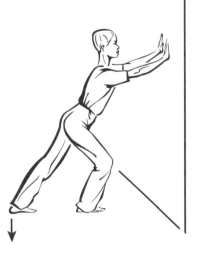

Combo 4: Leg Abductors (Outer Thighs)
Leg Raises

- Lie down on your side with your entire body in a straight line. Extend the arm nearest the floor out to the side for balance.
- Slowly lift one leg out to the side as high as possible, keeping the leg straight and in line with the hip. Keeping the foot pointed toward the nose, lift the leg over 4 seconds. Lower the leg back down to the starting position over 4 seconds.
- Repeat this movement 8 to 12 times then switch legs.

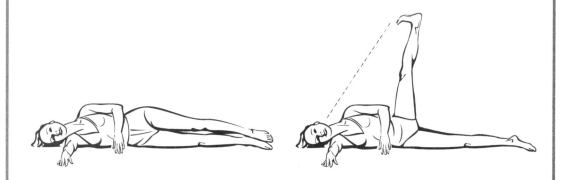

- Correcting form: The back should remain straight throughout the exercise.

Leg Stretches

- Stand with your feet shoulder width apart, knees slightly bent and stomach tight. Cross your right leg over your left leg.
- Bend at the hips, keeping the back straight, and reach down towards to the right until you feel a stretch. Hold for 15 to 30 seconds. Relax and repeat 8–12 times.
- Repeat on the other side.
- Correcting form: Watch for the back rounding. The back should be kept straight to maximize the stretch.

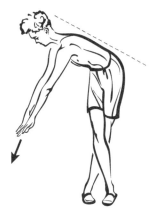

Combo 5: Gluteals (Buttocks)
Pelvic Raises

- Lie down on your back on a comfortable surface with your arms at your sides, palms down. Bend your knees to 90 degrees and keep your feet flat on the floor. This is your starting position.
- Over 4 seconds, raise your hips into the air by squeezing the muscles in the backs of your thighs and your buttocks. The aim is to make a straight line through your knees to your head. Try not to push on the floor with your hands. Only use your hands for balance.
- Now, lower your body back down to the starting position over 4 seconds.
- Repeat this exercise 8 to 12 times.
- Correcting form: The upper body should not be tensed during the entire movement.

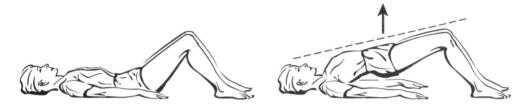

Buttocks Stretches

- Lie on your back, knees bent and feet flat on the floor. Cross the left leg over the right leg, resting the ankle of the left leg just above the right knee.
- Lift the right leg toward your chest and grab the back of the leg with both hands. Gently pull the left leg into the chest until you feel a stretch. Hold for 15 to 30 seconds.
- Repeat crossing the right leg.

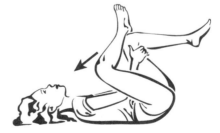

Combo 6: Rhomboids (Upper Back)
Bent-Over Rows

- Stand beside a bench or low table. Place the left knee on a bench and lean over to place the left palm on the bench under the left shoulder. Make sure the left elbow is not locked and the right arm hangs freely, right foot flat on the floor. This is your starting position.
- Keeping your back straight and parallel to the bench, slowly bring the right arm up, allowing the elbow to bend and pulling the right shoulder blade toward the middle of the back. This movement should take 2 to 4 seconds. Slowly return to the starting position over 2 to 4 seconds.
- Repeat this movement 8 to 12 times on each side.
- Increase the resistance by adding a small dumbbell or improvise using a can of soup.
- Correcting form: The upper body should remain in line with the bench. Correct rotation in the torso and sagging in the back.

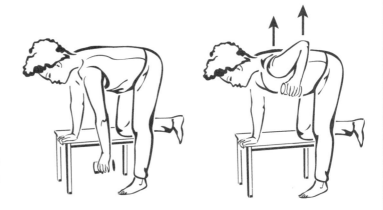

Upper Back Stretches

- Stand with your feet shoulder width apart. Keeping a slight bend in the knees, tuck your hips and tighten your stomach muscles. Bring your arms straight out in front of you, interlocking your fingers palms facing away from you.
- Round your upper back and allow your chin to fall onto your upper chest. Push your hands forward, feeling a stretch between your shoulder blades. Hold this stretch for 15 to 30 seconds.
- Relax and repeat.

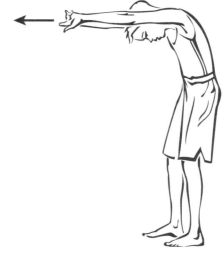

Combo 7: Pectorals (Chest Muscles)
Wall Push-Ups

- Stand straight with your legs shoulder-width apart at arm's length or greater from a wall. Lean forward and place your hands greater than shoulder width apart on the wall. This is your starting position.

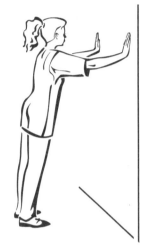
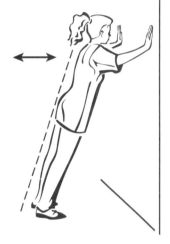

- Slowly bend your elbows and move your chest to the wall over 2 to 4 seconds. Now push with your hands and slowly return to the starting position over 2 to 4 seconds.
- Repeat 8 to 12 times.
- Correcting form: The legs should be straight during the entire movement but knees should not be locked. There should be a straight line from heals to head.

Chest Stretches

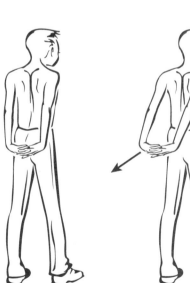

- Stand with your feet shoulder-width apart. Keep a slight bend in the knees, with stomach muscles tight. Reach your hands behind you and clasp your hands together palms in.
- Squeeze your elbows and shoulder blades together keeping your head, neck, and shoulders relaxed. Gently raise your arms back behind you. Hold this stretch for 15 to 30 seconds.
- Release the stretch and then repeat it one time.

Combo 8: Deltoids (Shoulders)
Lateral Arm Raises

- Stand straight and tall with your stomach muscles tight and your hips tight and slightly tucked. Now set your shoulder blades by shrugging your shoulders to your ears, squeezing them to the back and lowering them. Hold your shoulder blades there as you make fists. This is the starting position.
- Raise your fists up and out to the side over 2 to 4 seconds, finishing with your fists in line with your shoulders. Keep the arms straight but don't lock the elbows. Lower arms to the starting position over 2 to 4 seconds.
- Repeat 8 to 12 times.
- Increase the resistance by adding small dumbbells or improvise using cans of soup.
- Correcting form: Keep the stomach muscles tight and the back straight during the entire movement. Only the arms and shoulders should be moving.

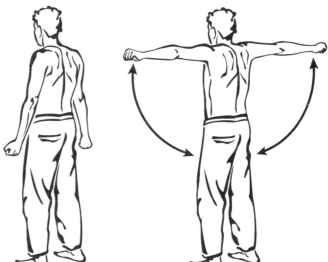

Shoulder Stretches

- Stand with your feet shoulder width apart. Keep a slight bend in the knees, with stomach muscles tight.
- Reach across your chest with your right arm. With your left hand grab your upper arm just above the elbow. Gently push your right arm towards your chest until you feel a stretch. Hold for 15 to 30 seconds. Relax and repeat.
- Repeat using the left arm.

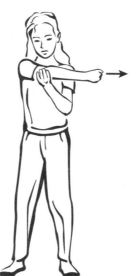

Combo 9: Biceps (Front of Upper Arms)
Biceps Curls

- Stand straight with feet shoulder width apart, keeping stomach muscles tight. Start by shrugging your shoulders as high as you can and squeezing your shoulder blades together. Lower you shoulders. This is the body position for the entire movement.
- With your arms at your sides, move your elbows snugly against your hips. This is your starting position.
- Slowly raise your fists over 4 seconds so that they almost reach your shoulders, keeping your elbows against your hips. Lower your fist back down to the starting position over 4 seconds.
- Repeat this movement 8 to 12 times for each arm.
- Increase resistance by adding small dumbells.
- Correcting form: The movement happens only at the elbow. Watch for any other movement during the exercise. There should be a straight line from heels to hips to shoulders to ears.

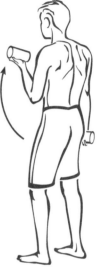

Biceps Stretches

- Stand straight with your stomach muscles tight and your feet shoulder width apart, knees slightly bent. Hold your arms out to the side, palms facing downward with thumbs pointing forward. Now point the thumbs toward the floor with palms facing backward. This is your starting position.
- From here, stretch the arms back so that the fingers are pointing toward the rear and a slight stretch is felt. Hold for 15 to 30 seconds.
- Repeat.

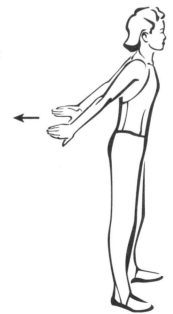

Combo 10: Triceps (Back of Upper Arms)
Triceps Dips

* Sit on a stable chair with your legs straight out in front of you and your feet together. Place your hands at your sides beside your hips. With your arms straight but elbows not locked, slide your hips forward so that you are a few inches in front of the edge of the chair. This is your starting position.
* Slowly lower yourself toward the ground by allowing your elbows to bend. Lower yourself 6 to 8 inches, pause, and then raise yourself back to the starting position.
* Correcting form: The elbows should be pointing back throughout the movement, not out to the side. Feet should remain relaxed through the movement. Shoulders should be held back and low, not shrugged up toward the ears.

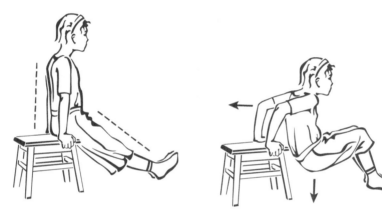

Tricep Stretches

* Stand with your feet shoulder width apart. Keep a slight bend in the knees and stomach muscles tight.
* Raise your right hand above your head, bend your elbow, and let your hand fall behind your head between your shoulder blades. Reach with your left hand and gently grasp your right elbow. Gently pull your right elbow toward your left side until you feel a stretch. Hold for 15 to 30 seconds. Relax and repeat twice.
* Repeat stretch for the right side.

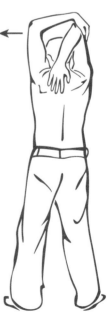

Combo 11: Lumbar (Lower Back)
Back Extensions

* Lie on your stomach on a comfortable surface. Bring your fingers to touch the sides of your head. This is your starting position.
* Gently begin to raise your shoulders 2 or 3 inches off the ground. As you do this, your head and arms will follow, but the neck should not arch backward. Imagine someone is pulling you up by strings attached to your shoulders.
* Raise your body slowly for 2 to 4 seconds and then slowly come back to the starting position over 4 seconds. Repeat this movement 8 to 12 times.
* Correcting form: The arms and legs should be relaxed during the entire exercise. The head should remain in line with the upper back. The movement should be slow and smooth.

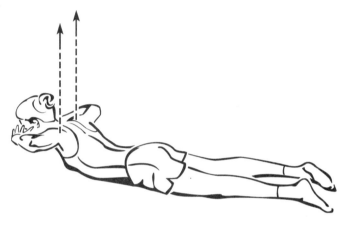

Lower Back Stretches

* Lie on your back on a comfortable surface relaxing your legs, back, arms, and head. Gently press your lower back toward the floor.
* Slowly bring both knees toward your chest and hold your legs behind the knees (not directly on the knee joint). Squeeze your legs into your chest until you feel a stretch. Hold for 15 to 30 seconds.
* Relax and repeat.

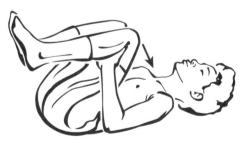

Combo 12: Stomach (Abdominals)
Stomach Crunches

- Lie on your back on a comfortable surface with your feet flat against a wall and your knees bent at 90 degrees. Rest your fingers gently behind your head. Press your lower back toward the floor. Keep the eyes focused on a spot high on the wall. This is your starting position.
- Squeeze your stomach muscles so that you are lifting your shoulders a few inches off the ground, toward the spot you are focusing on. This movement is slow, lasting 2 to 4 seconds.
- Keep your head and arms relaxed. You should not be pulling your head forward. To avoid squeezing your chin against your chest, imagine there is an orange between your chin and neck.
- When your shoulders are a few inches off the ground, hold this position for 1 second. Lower yourself back to the starting position over 4 seconds, feeling your stomach muscles contracting the whole way down. Repeat this movement 8 to 12 times.
- Correcting form: The movements should not be jerky. Watch for pulling on the neck, pushing the stomach out, and pushing the elbows forward.

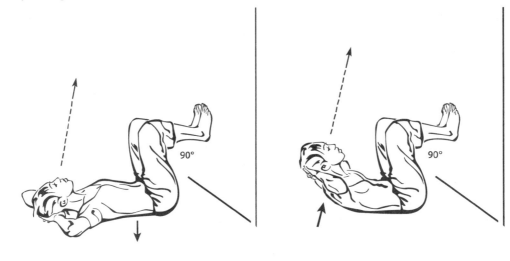

Abdominal Stretches

- Lie on your stomach on a comfortable surface. Place hands shoulder width apart, palms down, keeping your elbows close to your body.
- Push your upper body off the floor arching your back and keeping your lower body in contact with the floor. Do not lock your elbows.
- Repeat.

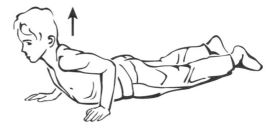

Choosing Enjoyable and Appropriate Activities

Different activities suit different bodies and personalities. When helping your child choose activities, it is important to keep in mind their physical abilities. This is especially important if your child is overweight and has been inactive. Many of the vigorous activities will be extremely difficult, if not impossible, for children who have a big discrepancy between their body weight and height or if they are physically unfit. While vigorous activity is the goal, some children need to start out a little slower than others, and progress may also be a little slower. Celebrating smaller successes and keeping the long-term goal in mind is important for building up and keeping lifelong habits of activity.

Not every endurance, strength, or flexibility activity will appeal to your child. Work with your child to select physical activities and sports they will enjoy. Just because you played the sport as a child doesn't mean your child will want to follow in your footsteps. If your child does not enjoy the activity or feels pressured to participate, the activity may become a chore and a bore. They will be less likely to continue on their own. Some imagination may be needed to find activities they like. Don't be afraid to experiment until you find a good fit.

Children also need to have some sense of personal control over the amount of time and effort they spend being active. Everyday opportunities for unplanned activity should always be sought, even if it is as simple as choosing to take the stairs instead of the escalator in the shopping mall, or washing the dishes instead of putting them in the dishwashing machine. Parents also need to be careful not to use activity as a punishment, either by forcing the child to do some activity they don't want to do or stopping them from doing some activity that they enjoy.

> ✔ **FACT**
>
> **Lifelong Pleasure**
> The goal is to keep your children active so that they might learn to enjoy the feeling and benefits of activity. Physical activity can then become a pleasurable, lifelong habit that maintains healthy weight and good health.

CASE STUDY Anne's Family

The 5-K Celebration

The morning was cool and a little cloudy as everyone milled about in front of the starting line. The nip of autumn was definitely in the air. Anne reminded Cody to take it slow, not start too fast, and walk a bit if he got too tired. She knew that Bill and Mark were out to compete with each other, Mark wanting to prove that he could "beat the old man." She would hang back and encourage Cody. Anne was nervous and wondered if she had done the right thing, but everyone seemed very excited and energized. The gun went off, and Bill and Mark were gone. She knew that they would be cheering for them when Cody crossed the finish line.

Cody started off great, a nice easy pace. She jogged along beside, and although people were passing them, they shouted encouragement as they went by. After the first kilometer, Cody wanted to go faster, so they picked it up a bit, but he gradually started slowing down. When they passed the 4-kilometer mark, Anne could tell he was getting tired, so she suggested they might walk for a minute. "No," Cody exclaimed, "I want to see if I can run the whole way."

In another 3 minutes they could see the crowd at the finish line and, to Anne's surprise, Cody started running faster. Soon, they could see Bill and Mark jumping up and down, and in a flash she grabbed Cody's hand as they bolted across the finish line. Cody started to cry, and so did Anne, but they were tears of joy and accomplishment. Bill and Mark ran up for a family group hug. They had done it, all of them!

Back at home, everyone had their own race story, even though they had all run the same race. Mark was boasting how he had sprinted ahead of his father. Bill laughed, "Don't be so sure next time!" Cody shouted, "Next time we do a 10-K!"

For lunch, Anne had baked lasagna, everyone's favorite. They cheered as they tucked in to their meal, no one complaining about the salad, or the fact that Anne had substituted half of the meat in the recipe with Mark's new favorite vegetable, eggplant. She also had used low-fat cheese and whole wheat noodles, but after their morning run, they were famished, and besides, it tasted great. The lasagna disappeared, and so did the salad. She then reached into the refrigerator and pulled out a chocolate angel food cake, a bowl of fresh blueberries and strawberries, and a container of fat-free lemon yogurt. They cheered again. Dessert for lunch!

At his next checkup, Cody's doctor was impressed. While Cody was still a long way from his ideal weight, he had lost 9 pounds over the last 6 months. His cholesterol level and liver tests were much better, and he seemed to be happier. Cody bragged to the doctor about how he had run a 5-K race, and that maybe next year he would try a 10-K race. He suggested that the doctor might give it a try. The doctor and Anne laughed. "Maybe my mom could help you, too," Cody exclaimed. "Thinking about starting your own clinic, Anne?" the doctor teased. "My family's health is my priority and my success story, and I plan to keep it that way," she replied.

Fit Tips

- Encourage young children to help with household chores. Most young people like to help out.

- Encourage older children to be involved in the promotion of physical activities for other kids at school or even in the community.

- Give your children toys, games, and sports equipment for birthday or holiday presents that will increase their physical activity.

- After sitting in school all day, children should play when they first get home instead of watching television or doing homework.

- Enroll your children in age-appropriate and developmentally appropriate sports and recreational activities.

- If your child seems to be slow some days, offer them a choice among various moderate physical activities but do not permit them to be couch potatoes.

- Allow your child to be involved in as many different types of activities as possible so they can discover the ones they prefer.

- Ensure that new activities are introduced in non-threatening environments.

- Avoid drawing attention to your children's sedentary behavior; instead, praise your children often when they choose to be active

- Avoid imposing adult standards of physical activity on your child. An hour of active play is more appropriate for young children than running for an hour.

- Rubber band exercises can be great for children because the bands are relatively inexpensive, can be taken anywhere, and are a safer way to add resistance to exercises.

- Exercise balls can be a lot of fun for adults and kids alike. The exercises that can be performed using the ball can help your child develop strength, flexibility, and balance.

The Healthy Weight Program

The Healthy Weight Program described in the next chapter provides methods for encouraging physical activity by setting weekly activity goals. We offer an extensive list of MET-rated activities your child can choose from, as well as a record-keeping system to monitor progress in creating energy balance and getting a healthy weight through physical activity.

CHAPTER 8

The Healthy Weight Program

With a solid understanding of the role of good nutrition and physical activity in getting and keeping a healthy weight for your child, we can set out a program for you and your child to follow. If you have read the previous chapters in this book, you will have all of the knowledge that you will need to help your child take the first steps toward a healthy weight. However, even if you have not read the previous chapters in this book you can still begin the program. You can always go back and read other parts of the book when you have questions. Reading the first chapters of this book will give you a better understanding of how your child may have become overweight and how the program works to reverse that trend.

CASE STUDY Andrea's Program

Breathless

"C'mon girls!" Anna, the dance teacher yelled. "Just hold the stretch for 3 more seconds." Andrea felt her face turn red as she struggled to hold the stretch. Sweat was pouring down her face as she continued to listen to Anna. It had only been 5 minutes into the class and she was already overcome with a shortness of breath. Andrea quickly moved to the back of the room hoping that no one else had seen her struggle.

How could she have let her friend Robyn convince her to take part in the after-school dance class? This was an awful decision. Andrea decided that it was best if she continued to follow the class from the back row so that no one else could see her difficulties. All of Andrea's friends eagerly participated next to the dance teacher but her embarrassment would not allow her to do this. Andrea had never really thought that her weight was an issue, though this was affecting her ability to keep up in dance class.

"Ok!" she told herself, "only 20 more minutes until this horror is over." She felt so out of shape watching the other girls easily participating in the dance class as she had to struggle to keep herself motivated. She did not want this to continue. She needed to get a healthier weight and become more active.

continued on page 230

Program Philosophy

Your child will take small manageable steps toward healthy nutrition and healthy activity habits by choosing weekly nutrition and activity goals. By taking these steps, your child will start having a healthy lifestyle and will become physically fit and get a healthy weight.

Starting the Program

Regardless of your children's age when they start this program, you will be facing the difficult task of trying to undo what may be years of poor eating habits and activity patterns. This may be true for you and your whole family. You will be asking your child, yourself, and your family to cut back on less healthy food choices and to increase healthy alternatives. You will also be asking your children to change their physical activity habits by becoming more active. This may involve changing such deep-rooted habits as watching television after school or playing computer games in the evening.

Family Support

A supportive family environment will be necessary to help your child develop a healthier lifestyle and get to a healthy weight. You and your family already serve as examples that affect your child's eating and activity habits. The participation of the whole family in the program will guarantee the greatest success. Eating healthy and being active is important for everyone's health, even family members who may already be at a healthy weight. When the whole family joins in the program, your child will not feel singled out and everyone becomes healthier.

Food Changes

The most effective way to improve your family's nutrition is to improve the food environment at home. Doing this will take some time, and your family may be unwilling to make these changes at the beginning. Introducing healthier nutrition to your child and your family should not involve complete restriction of any foods. Instead, the focus should be on decreasing how much and how often less healthy foods are available, and looking for healthier alternatives that your child and your family enjoy. The changes you make will need to be small and spread out over a long period of time.

Healthy Weight

This is the weight your child's body reaches with healthy nutrition and healthy activity habits. That weight will be different for each child and there is no one particular number that your child needs to reach. If your child is living a healthy lifestyle, their body will find its own healthy weight.

Food Environment

This is an important part for improving your child's health. You and your child will use the program to help build a healthier food environment at home and away from home. The grocery store tour in this book teaches you about better food choices. It is your responsibility as a concerned parent to increase the number of healthy foods you make available in your home and decrease the less healthy ones.

Q: **How do I handle my child's food environment outside the home?**

A: Your child spends a large amount of time in food environments that you may feel are beyond your reach. School is one such place. At school, being the only child in class without the latest chocolate or candy snack can leave your child feeling deprived. They may even be teased.

Restricting all less healthy snack foods may only make them more desirable because they are forbidden and increase the likelihood that your child will eat them when you are not around. Restricting less healthy snack foods in the house but allowing them once in a while outside the home, such as at school, is a good plan.

Food Preparation

Making healthy foods a main concern in your home makes it easier to prepare foods that are more nutritious and more filling for your child and family. Your responsibility is to incorporate healthier food preparation into your family's meals by encouraging all family members to chip in and by giving them options from among the various groups of wholesome foods.

Food Choices

Teaching your child about nutrition will make it easier for them to understand what healthier food choices are. They will be able to use what they have learned to make healthier food choices in the home, at school, at friend's houses, and even on occasional visits to a restaurant or fast-food outlet.

Physical Activity Changes

Increasing the amount of activity in your child's daily routine is a trial and error process. It may be hard to change old habits, such as sitting in front of the television or computer after school. You should expect that increasing your child's activity levels will be a gradual process with some stalling and setbacks along the way.

Family Exercise Routine

The best plan for increasing your child's activity level is by involving the whole family. Having regular and planned family activities will increase the chances that the family gets in the good habit of being active. These activities could include family walks after dinner on most days or weekend trips to the parks. Finding enjoyable activities will make sure that the whole family wants to play a part.

When introducing a new activity to your family and your child, the first step will be to make the activity a habit or routine. Your family and child need to build new activities into their normal schedule and to expect to be doing them regularly. Once new activities are routine, then the focus can be on the amount of activity.

Parent participation in physical activities is necessary for children to want to stay involved. Studies show that children of parents who are active are more likely to be active themselves when they grow up. Children of inactive parents are more likely to grow up to be inactive as adults.

> **Physically Fit**
>
> When children are physically fit, they will be able to complete the program's recommended amounts of physical activity without being physically uncomfortable, without having difficulty breathing, and without getting tired during and being overly tired afterward.

Q: **What do I do if my child complains about taking part in an activity?**

A: Listen to your children. If they are participating in an activity and say they are tired or hurting, they probably are. Young people are not as likely to continue with physical activity if they are tired while doing it, if it is boring or if it makes them uncomfortable. If any of these are true, find more enjoyable choices.

Make sure that you are also sensitive to other reasons why they may be complaining about an activity. Are they lacking confidence in their abilities? Are other children teasing them? Have they had a bad experience before with a particular activity? Be sure to look at all of the possible reasons why your child may not wish to take part in a particular activity. If these reasons remain hidden, they can have long lasting effects on your child's willingness to take part in the activity or similar activities.

Parent's Role in the Program: Do's and Don'ts

DO:

Be an Effective Role Model or a Good Example: When you are physically active, your child is more likely to be physically active. Find activities that you are comfortable participating in and have your child join you.

Be a Fan: When your child gets praise and positive feedback while they are being active, they are much more likely to keep going with the activity. When we have fans cheering us on, we often become more energized and try harder. Offer encouragement to your child whenever they take part in any sort of activity.

Be a Coach: Show interest in your child's activities. Help them find activities they enjoy or do extremely well at. Frequently check how they are doing and make sure they have the proper equipment. Help them to get the skills they need to take part fully. Make charts and records of their successes. Go watch them play.

Be a Proud Parent: Show enthusiasm and give appropriate rewards. Take pictures of your child while they are being active or make signs and banners and put them on the fridge. Mention your child's successes to your friends while your child is around and able to hear.

Be a Leader: Get involved with your child's school and/or community activity programs. Get connected with other parents at school and try to influence the school for more physical activity opportunities. Get together with neighbors and start a regular group activity plan for all the children on your street. If you see an opportunity for starting a new activity in the community, volunteer to help.

Be a Chaperone or Chauffeur: Walk your child and other children in the neighborhood to places where they will be physically active. When necessary, provide transportation to community centers or other locations of physical activity. Share the responsibility with other parents in your neighborhood. There may be opportunities for your child to become friends with other children who are physically active.

Be Creative: Organized sports are great, but it is just as important to help your child find ways to be active in and around the home, and by themselves. Get your children involved in weekly chores. Also, find creative ways of encouraging physical activity, such as making a room in the house the active playroom. Look for presents and rewards that encourage active play outside the home, such as skipping ropes, Frisbees, balls and racquets.

DON'T:

Criticize: Criticizing your child about their poor eating choices or their lack of activity will often backfire and could lead them to resent healthier eating and physical activity. Instead, praise and applaud them when they make healthier food choices and when they get involved in any physical activity. Always offer healthy options to less healthy food choices and periods of inactivity, but never criticize.

Discourage: It may seem obvious but it is easy to be unaware of how some comments can be discouraging and sometimes hurtful for children. For example, if your child overhears you telling your friend about how your child is always eating less healthy food or is lazy, it can be very upsetting. As their parent, you must support your child. Praise them and bring to everyone's attention the healthy behaviors of your child and try not to pay as much attention to the less healthy behaviors. The attention that the healthy behaviors get will go a long way toward encouraging more of the same.

Nag: Constantly nagging your child about what they are eating or about being inactive will not help them to change. Imagine how you feel when you are nagged or harassed by others.

Blame: Children are not directly responsible for their weight, their food choices or their activity habits. All of these things come from their environment and from their genes. Their environment is partly controlled by you and your family. Children can learn eating and activity habits from the family. The foods that they eat the most are clearly determined by which foods the family keeps in the house. The time they spend watching television and on the computer is also determined by what the family allows. The family's level of activity partly determines whether your child will be active or inactive. Because your child's eating and activity habits are most often determined by conditions they have never had any direct control over, it is never proper to blame them.

Tease: Teasing doesn't just come from other children, but can come from adults and family members as well. Teasing will not make your child more interested in healthy behavior. Teasing from other family members or children at school should not be tolerated.

Restrict: Research shows that completely restricting foods only increases their appeal and the likelihood that your child will want to have the restricted foods, particularly when you are not around. Instead of strictly limiting some foods, focus on decreasing the amount of those foods that are available to be eaten. You may choose to limit the types of foods you keep in your house, and instead make special trips or create special occasions for eating those foods outside the house. Restricting physical activity, unfortunately, does not have the same effect of increasing its appeal, and only results in decreasing further the amount of energy your child uses up in the day. Punishments should not involve limiting opportunities for physical activity or particular foods.

continued on next page

DON'T:

Use Food as a Reward: Food is all too commonly used as a reward these days, especially less healthy foods. Parents soothe their children with sweet snacks, they limit dessert until dinner is eaten and the plate is clean, and they use treats as presents. In these cases, children can begin to see the less healthy snacks as more pleasing and healthy foods as less tasty and less attractive. It can be very difficult for families to change their habit of using food as a reward because most of us grew up viewing some foods in this way. Food has been a way that some parents express love and caring. In some cases, parents feel guilty that they have less time to spend with their children because they work long hours. When you wish to give your children more than praise for their accomplishments, or just to show that you are thinking about them, choose non-food rewards, such as toys, sports equipment, stickers, or tickets to some event.

Be Inconsistent: Children need boundaries and limits. This also applies to their behavior around food and activity. Stick to whatever boundaries and limits you set. If you decide as a family that the television should not be turned on during dinner, be consistent with this decision. Limits and boundaries should also be set equally for all members of the family, including parents. Sometimes there may be a legitimate excuse for a difference, but a healthy weight is not an excuse for siblings or parents to eat less healthy and be less active.

Show Favoritism: You may have already found yourself treating your overweight child differently than their siblings. This can cause your child to feel guilty and responsible for their less healthy body weight. Try not to single out one child while making changes to the food available for everyone. For example, it is not okay to feed your family chocolate cake for dessert but not to allow one child to have any.

Do as I Say, Not as I Do: Asking your child to eat healthier and be more active is far less successful if you yourself don't do so. Your children will find it much easier to change their habits if others in the family are making the same attempts. Be sure that you are trying to improve your own nutrition and physical activity levels at the same time as your child.

Lie or Trick: These are always poor approaches with children. Children can often tell when we are lying or tricking them, and when they do figure it out, we lose all trustworthiness. We encourage you to be creative in finding helpful ways of encouraging healthy behavior, without resorting to tricking or deceiving your children.

Punish: Don't use punishment (or threats of punishment) to try and change your child's eating and activity habits. Punishing children for less healthy eating or lack of physical activity is not a successful strategy for teaching anyone to enjoy eating nutritiously or being physically active. Threatening to take away dessert because your child is misbehaving teaches the same improper relationship to food as does rewarding them with food, and makes those less healthy foods more wanted. Threatening to increase the amount or types of physical activity your child performs as a punishment will make those activities seem like punishment at other times and make them less enjoyable.

Q: **How long will it take before we see changes?**

A: Children do not become overweight overnight. Most often, it happens without parents noticing, until one day, a comment is made to them or to the child by another family member, friend, or a doctor. Similarly, helping children to get a healthy weight is a slow process and requires a lot of patience.

Each child who follows our program will be at a different starting point. They may be at a different weight, at a different stage of development, and at unique nutrition and physical activity levels. Also, each person's genetics determines how their body reacts to the food that they eat and to their level of physical activity. For these reasons, it is difficult to determine an exact time frame for the program.

General Time Line for Change

1 Month
Often it takes at least a month for new behaviors to become automatic or routine — for example, remembering to eat fruit at breakfast each day without being told or automatically choosing to take the stairs instead of an escalator. The healthy weight program presented here focuses on the first crucial month for changing old and strengthening new nutrition and activity habits.

3 Months
It can take up to 3 months before your child's body starts making longer lasting changes in the way it responds to physical activity. If you and your child follow the program, you can expect to see important changes in your child's eating and activity habits after 3 months, but probably even sooner. Taking part in physical activity should also be less difficult and more desirable for your child.

6 Months
Your children will have good physical fitness, and they may start to look more healthy and fit as well.

1 Year
If the efforts have been consistent, your child will be physically fit. It may be hard to imagine right now, but they will be fit as long as they follow the guidelines for nutrition and physical activity set out in the program.

Beyond a Year

Even though your child will be fit after a year, they may not yet be at a completely healthy weight. Their body may need more time. It will depend on your child's level of overweight when they started the program. They will eventually reach a healthy weight though, because the program is designed to help your child make permanent and lasting lifestyle changes.

Weight-Loss Factors

Muscle Weight

Your children's changes in height during the time they are working with the program will have a big effect on the changes you will see in their weight. With increased height comes increased muscle and water in the body. Muscle and water both weigh more than body fat. Because of this, you cannot rely too much on the number on the weigh scale. For example, if your child grew about 1 inch over a period of a few months, the extra muscle and water would weigh around 5 pounds. In this case, your child may not have been adding body fat and may even have been losing it, but because of the extra muscle and water, the weight on the scale wouldn't show it.

In addition, as children become more physically active, especially as they begin and move through puberty and beyond, they may build up more muscle. Strong muscles weigh more. Boys will accumulate more than girls. This is another reason why the weight from the scale may not be a true measure of body fat.

Q: **Why do fad diets seem to work faster than The Healthy Weight Program?**

A: This program is not a diet, nor is it like the fad diets and programs promoted for adults. Those diets and programs often claim rapid weight loss and endorse changes in food choices that are impossible to keep going for long. Those programs for adults most often fail. For children, those types of programs for adults often involve dietary changes that may be unsafe. The nutrition and activity goals of our program are based on American and Canadian governmental health recommendations. As children meet the goals set out by this program, they will be headed toward a healthy weight and toward becoming healthier.

Body Shape Changes

The changes that happen in your child's body shape when they start the program may be hard for you and your child to notice. The changes may only be noticed by relatives and friends who have not seen your child for some time. It may be useful for you to take pictures of your child every so often so that it will be easier to see the changes that are happening.

A Healthy Weight

Health cannot be measured on a scale.

The most important message you can give to your child is that the goal is not to lose a lot of weight. The goal of this program is to have good nutrition and to develop an active lifestyle. As young people move closer to the eating habits and physical activity levels within the program, their body's will naturally develop a healthy weight in a healthy amount of time.

Healthy lifestyle can be measured.

A healthy lifestyle is a lifestyle where nutritious food is eaten on a regular basis and an important amount of physical activity is performed each day. The program provides the way to measure and record if your child is eating nutritiously and if they are getting a healthy amount of physical activity. Seeing improvements in eating habits and activity levels will give your child encouragement and a sense of accomplishment in the first weeks of the program when changes in weight and appearance may not be seen.

Program Levels

Your child will take small steps toward healthy nutrition and healthy activity habits by choosing weekly nutrition and activity goals. By taking these steps, your child will start accepting a healthy lifestyle and will become physically fit and get to a healthy weight.

The program has a series of levels leading up to healthy nutrition and activity habits. These levels clearly show how well your child is doing with their nutrition and activity level.

At the First Steps level, your child is at the very beginning of the road to healthy nutrition or activity. From here, the levels go from Copper, through Bronze and Silver to Gold. The Gold level is difficult for most children to keep going at every single day, but it should be the goal for most days of the week. At the Gold level, all of the recommendations we have made for healthy nutrition and healthy activity habits are met most days of the week.

- **First Steps:** Your child is at the beginning of the road to healthy nutrition and activity.
- **Copper:** Your child is on the way to a healthy active lifestyle.
- **Bronze:** Your child is close to reasonably healthy nutrition and activity habits.
- **Silver:** Your child is doing very well and has good nutrition and physical activity habits.
- **Gold:** Your child is meeting all the recommendations for nutrition and physical activity and is living a very healthy active lifestyle.

Gold Level Nutrition Goals

Healthy nutrition means that your child is getting an adequate amount of wholesome foods, including vegetables, fruit, whole grain foods, legumes, fish, poultry, eggs, lean meat, and adequate amounts of calcium. It also means that your child chooses to limit the amount of processed foods in the diet, such as refined starches, sugar, soft drinks/fruit drinks, and saturated fat. Levels have been determined for each of these categories.

The gold level recommendations for the daily amount to eat in each category of nutrition are shown here. One serving is a specific amount of food. The amount depends on its food group. When you start the program, you will learn how to decide how many servings your child has eaten from each food category.

Your child will aim to reach these Gold levels on most days of the week.

Gold Level Nutrition	
Wholesome Foods	**Daily Amount**
Vegetables	More than 5 servings
Fruit	3 servings
Whole Grain	5 or more servings
Legumes/Nuts	2 servings
Fish, Poultry, Eggs, Lean Meat	2-3 servings
Calcium Source	3 servings (4-8 yrs)/4 servings (9-18 yrs)
Processed Foods	**Daily Amount**
Refined Starches	1 serving or none
Sweet Drinks/Juice	1 cup (250 ml) or less
Other foods high in sugar and saturated fat	Keep to a minimum

Gold Level Activity Habits

Healthy activity means that your child participates in moderate and vigorous physical activity on a daily basis. Part of healthy activity habits also mean that your child intends to limit their screen time (television, video games, computer games, surfing the internet for fun). Performing strength and stretching exercises on two days of each week is also a healthy habit for your child to develop.

The Gold level recommendations for each category of daily activity are shown here. Moderate physical activity includes walking from place to place or leisurely bike rides. In moderate activity, a person is breathing faster but can usually carry on a normal conversation.

Vigorous physical activity includes jogging and other fast-paced activities. In vigorous activity, a person is breathing deeply and rapidly and would find it difficult to carry on a normal conversation.

Your child will aim to reach the Gold level on most days of the week.

Gold Level Activity	
Activity	**Amount per Day**
Moderate Physical Activity	60 minutes
Vigorous Physical Activity	30 minutes
Screen Time	Limit to 1 hour maximum

Weekly Program Goals

Each week, with your help, your child will choose one nutrition goal and one activity goal from a list of program goals we have provided. The nutrition and activity goals can be either knowledge goals or action goals:

- **Knowledge Goals:** These goals aim to teach each your child something important about nutrition or physical activity.
- **Action Goals:** These goals aim to change something about your child's nutrition or physical activity that should bring your child to a higher program level for one category of nutrition or activity habits.

These goals can be custom-made to balance, individualize, or go beyond the standard program's knowledge and activity goals for nutrition and physical activity.

Here are examples of nutrition and activity program goals for a week and examples of specific personalized goals your child might set to complete them:

Nutrition: Action
Program Goal: Eat more fruit this week.
Personalized Goal: Eat one apple for breakfast on Monday,
Wednesday, and Friday.

Nutrition: Knowledge
Program Goal: Learn how to read nutrition labels.
Personalized Goal: Go shopping with mom and find a break-
fast cereal I think I'll like that is low in sugar.

Activity: Action
Program Goal: Run a 3-km race.
Personalized Goal: Jog around the block for 5 minutes on
Monday and Wednesday right after school.

Activity: Knowledge
Program Goal: Participate in a team or individual sport.
Personalized Goal: On Tuesday after school I will go with
Dad to the community center to look for a sport that I would
like to get involved in.

Keeping Records

Three months is a long time for a child or an adult to have to
wait to see changes. That is one of the reasons that it is so
important to keep records of the smaller changes your child
is making. This will help you and your child become aware of
small improvements each week, even if weight, body shape
and fitness take longer to change. A wide variety of record-
keeping forms are provided in this program.

Keeping records in the program will require a small
amount of time from you and your child, especially when
you are first learning. During the first few months before
physical changes are obvious, the records of small successes
will be a key source of encouragement and will help your
child to stay motivated to keep going with the program. The
extra few minutes you spend helping your child now will
result in changes that may last a lifetime. Remember that
the main focus of the program is your child's health, meaning healthy eating and activity habits, not weight number on
the scale.

Importance of Keeping Records

Staying on Track

By keeping records from time to time, you and your child will have a better picture of their nutrition and activity habits. The records will help highlight the specific areas of nutrition and physical activity that need to be improved so that they can focus on them. Keeping records also allows you to compare more recent records with older ones so that you can see when positive changes are occurring.

Improving Motivation

Seeing and praising changes, even the smallest ones, can be a great source of motivation for your children and help them to stick with the changes they are making. Often when people begin to record their food intake and become aware of it, they automatically change their habits for the better. Your child's weight may not change much at first, especially if they are growing quickly. Keeping records of nutrition, activity, and goals accomplished allows everyone to see all the great progress they are making instead of just focusing on losing weight. Seeing these changes can motivate them to continue with the program even during the times when their weight may not be changing.

Appreciating Accomplishments

By keeping track of changes in nutrition and activity, you will be able to give additional praise and encouragement, which is a very big motivator for children. Recognition of successes, no matter how small, is extremely important for a child's self-esteem. Using this program, your child will learn how to set goals and have a greater sense of control over how they progress through the program. They will feel that the program is their own. As they reach their set goals again and again, their self-confidence will improve.

Determining Rewards

Sometimes giving rewards can give your children the extra encouragement that they need to accomplish the more difficult goals. Be sure to give your children lots of praise while they are attempting their to meet their goals and beyond. Focus on all the positives and offer support for any unsuccessful attempts. Record-keeping can help you find out when your child has earned a reward. You will learn about suitable rewards in the program.

Program Records

Nutrition and Activity Levels

Using the worksheets we provide, your children will keep a food and activity diary from time to time while working through the program. With your help, they will use their diary to determine what program level they are at (Copper to Gold) as they begin to develop healthier eating and activity habits.

Weekly Goals

Weekly nutrition and activity goals will be recorded on the worksheets shown in this book and kept in a place where they can be seen so that your child is reminded about them throughout the week.

Height and Weight Measurements

Using the charts we provide, you will help your children measure and mark down their height and weight probably no more than once every 2 weeks.

Q: How long will we need to keep track of progress in the program?

A: Your child will not have to keep track of progress and set weekly goals forever. The program is meant to help your child build up lifelong healthy nutrition and activity habits. Every family will begin this program at a different starting level, and each child will get to a healthy body weight in a different amount of time. You can expect that establishing some habits will be easier for your child and your family than others. Some may take only weeks to develop, such as eating fruit on a daily basis; others may take several months, such as getting enough moderate and vigorous physical activity. It will be up to you and your child to decide when they are ready to put the program aside. They will be able carry on where they left off if they need a refresher in the future or have fallen off track.

However long you or your child remain on the program, the aim is to make healthy eating and physical activity a lifelong habit or routine. There are several good reasons why setting up routines is important for their success with the program. When a routine is in place, it will be much easier for parents and children to remember to complete the various records in the program. For example, you may decide that at a specific time each night, you will spend a few minutes with your child to go over their goals for the day or the week ahead, to discuss any difficulties or problems that they are having, and to complete program charts and diaries. This might also be a time for extra praise and to set rewards for your child's efforts. You may set other routines, such as family walks, walking or biking to school, or turning off the television at dinner. It will be easier for your child to take on healthier behaviors when they are part of a family routine that is predictable and expected.

Program Stages

The Healthy Weight Program follows four stages: assessment or finding the starting point, implementation or getting started, consolidation or doing it, and maintenance or keeping it going. Parent and child have particular knowledge and activity goals in each stage.

STAGE 1
Assessing Nutrition and Activity Levels (Week 1)
☐ Family Nutrition and Activity Habits Worksheet
☐ Child's Nutrition and Activity Habits Worksheet
☐ 3-Day Nutrition Diary: Log and Scorecard
☐ 3-Day Activity Diary: Log and Scorecard
☐ Height, Weight, and Target Weight Chart

STAGE 2
Setting Goals and Rewards (Week 2)
☐ Goal of the Week Worksheet
☐ Goal of the Week Evaluation Questionnaire
☐ 3-Day Nutrition Diary: Log and Scorecard
☐ 3-Day Activity Diary: Log and Scorecard

STAGE 3
Building Up Goals and Rewards (Week 3-4)
☐ Goal of the Week Worksheet
☐ Goal of the Week Evaluation Questionnaire
☐ 3-Day Nutrition Diary: Log and Scorecard
☐ 3-Day Activity Diary: Log and Scorecard
☐ Height, Weight, and Target Weight Chart

STAGE 4
Maintaining Progress (Beyond Week 4)
Weekly
☐ Goal of the Week Worksheet
☐ Goal of the Week Evaluation Questionnaire

Monthly
☐ 3-Day Nutrition Diary: Log and Scorecard
☐ 3-Day Activity Diary: Log and Scorecard
☐ Family Nutrition and Activity Habits Worksheet
☐ Child's Nutrition and Activity Habits Worksheet

Biweekly (Every 2 Weeks)
☐ Height, Weight, and Target Weight Chart

CASE STUDY Andrea's Program

Where am I?

Miss Nelson had been Andrea's teacher last semester for gym class. Andrea felt a little uneasy about approaching Miss Nelson about her weight problem, but the memory of her bad day in dance class helped push her to make a visit to Miss Nelson's office. Miss Nelson was enthusiastic about helping Andrea make healthy changes and asked her to come back during lunch hour so they could talk. After leaving the office, Andrea breathed a sigh of relief — asking for help was hard but she felt better.

During their lunch time appointment Miss Nelson showed Andrea a body mass index chart or BMI chart. She explained that this would help Andrea understand where her current weight was relative to what a healthy weight was for other 13-year-old girls that were her height. Miss Nelson stressed that there was a healthy range that Andrea should be aiming for. Miss Nelson weighed Andrea at 61 kilograms (135 pounds) and measured her height at 150 centimeters. Miss Nelson then showed Andrea how to calculate her BMI, which was 27.1. On the chart, this showed Andrea was over the 95th percentile for her age. Andrea was feeling discouraged. She had suspected that she weighed more than she should but had been able to brush it aside until now.

continued on page 235

STAGE 1

Assessing Nutrition and Activity Levels (Week 1)

The one-week assessment stage requires that you and your child keep records on a daily basis. This will help you to find out how your child is currently doing and where they are at concerning living a healthy lifestyle before they start using the program. This will take some effort, especially at the beginning. You will want to start the assessment when you know that you will be able to keep records on a daily basis for an entire week. Remember, this program is a long-term solution to helping your child achieve a healthy weight.

During the assessment stage of the program, do not make any efforts at changing your child's eating habits or activity level. The goal of the assessment is to get a true picture of your child's current eating habits and activity levels in order to find out their specific needs and to set goals. Treat the assessment seriously but not too seriously, so that your child does not feel like you are asking them to pass some sort of test. Also, if possible, have your child learn to use the records themselves under your guidance.

Young people should take responsibility for their nutrition and activity program over time. By involving them as much as possible in the record-keeping, they will be learning more about nutrition and physical activity.

Q: **When should we start the program?**

A: Starting the program when outside circumstances are going to make things more challenging is not ideal. For example, holidays, family trips and other events that are outside your child's normal routine will be less ideal times to do the assessment stage and to start the program. We do recommend that the starting date be a Monday so that the last day is the Sunday, a day when there may be a little more time to go over the results of the assessment.

Getting Started

By now, you are probably eager to get going and you probably want to start setting goals and making changes immediately in order to make a difference to your child's health. Let's begin by going over your child's current nutrition and activity habits and by completing a set of assessment worksheets to use as standards while watching your child's progress in the program. Learning how to use these worksheets may take some practice, but they will become easy to use very quickly. During this assessment stage, your child will have less involvement with using the program materials.

Stage 1 Preview (Week 1)

- ☐ Family Nutrition and Activity Habits Worksheet
- ☐ Child's Nutrition and Activity Habits Worksheet
- ☐ 3-Day Nutrition Diary: Log and Scorecard
- ☐ 3-Day Activity Diary: Log and Scorecard
- ☐ Height, Weight, and Target Weight Chart

Family Nutrition and Activity Habits Worksheet

This worksheet will allow you to measure your family's eating and exercise habits. We recommend that parents complete this worksheet now and every month during the program, so you might want to make some copies of the worksheet for future use. You can also come back to the worksheets to see how much progress is made from month to month.

Instructions

1. Check off all of the following statements about nutrition and activity that are currently true for you and your family.
2. After using the program for several months, you should agree with most of the statements.

Home Nutrition Behavior

☐ We use mostly low-fat cooking methods (e.g., baking, grilling, broiling, stir-frying).
☐ We eat together as a family on most days of the week.
☐ We don't eat dinner while watching television.
☐ We don't use food as a reward in any situation.

Home Kitchen (check your kitchen right now)

☐ Fresh fruit and/or vegetables are in the refrigerator and ready for snacking on.
☐ All of the packaged foods in our cupboards are free of trans fat and hydrogenated oils.
☐ Low-fat snacks are available (e.g., pretzels, air-popped popcorn).
☐ Healthy fat snacks are available (e.g., raw nuts, trail mix) in small amounts ($1/4$ cup).

Shopping Habits

☐ Fruit and vegetables take up the biggest amount of space in our shopping cart.
☐ All juice in the refrigerator is 100% pure juice.
☐ We try new/different vegetables that become available.
☐ We try new/different fruit varieties that become available.
☐ We choose whole-grain foods more often.
☐ We choose foods that are higher in fiber.
☐ When buying dairy products, we choose the lower-fat alternatives.
☐ When buying meat, we choose the lean varieties.
☐ We include fish in our family's diet.
☐ We include skinless chicken breast in our family's diet.
☐ We include meat alternatives in our family's diet (including lentils, beans and soy or tofu products).
☐ We make a point of buying foods that are low in saturated fat.
☐ We look at food labels and compare the nutrition of different products.
☐ We avoid buying products with trans fats.

Family Activity Habits

☐ We make time to do some kind of physical activity as a family at least once a week.
☐ Every member of the family takes part in regular physical activity each day (this could be as simple as going on a half-hour family walk each day).
☐ Every member of the family considers physical activity as enjoyable and not a chore.

Child's Nutrition and Activity Habits Worksheet

This worksheet will help you to measure your child's eating and exercise habits. We recommend that a parent and child complete this worksheet now and every month during the program, so you might want to make several copies of the worksheet for future use. You can also come back to the worksheets to see how much progress is made from month-to-month.

Instructions

1. Check off the following statements about nutrition and activity that are currently true for your child.
2. After using the program for several months, you should agree with most of the statements.

Child's Nutrition

☐ My child eats at fast-food restaurants (or orders in) no more than once every 2 weeks.
☐ My child drinks soft drinks/fruit drinks only once a week or less.
☐ My child eats chips or nachos only once a week or less.
☐ My child eats breakfast every single day.
☐ My child eats vegetables every single day.
☐ My child eats fruit every single day.
☐ My child doesn't eat meals or snacks in front of the television.
☐ My child is not restricted from eating foods that other family members eat.
☐ My child does not eat just because they are bored.
☐ My child does not eat just because they are upset.

Child's Activity Habits

☐ My child does not have a television, video games or computer in the bedroom.
☐ My child helps with activities and chores around the house, such as carrying the groceries, vacuuming, raking leaves or shoveling snow.
☐ My child wears appropriate safety equipment (helmet, mouth guard, eyewear) when taking part in activities.
☐ My child is not singled out as needing more physical activity.
☐ My child takes the stairs instead of using escalators and elevators.
☐ My child walks to school when possible.
☐ My child has a room in the house reserved for physical activity and play.

Estimating Nutrition Levels

Before completely assessing the nutrition and activity levels of your child, you might try estimating these levels. Using this chart, make a guess as to the number of servings you think your child eats of each food type. Don't worry about the definition of a serving size now. Just go by what you would normally serve in each category. We'll give you a chart for determining the serving size of various food types later.

Nutrition Level Estimate		
Type of Food	**Recommended Gold Level Daily Servings**	**Your Guess**
Wholesome Foods		
Vegetables	6 or more	
Fruit	3	
Whole Grains	5 or more	
Legumes, Nuts, Seeds	2	
Fish, Poultry, Eggs, Lean Meat	2-3	
Calcium Sources	3-4	
Processed Foods		
Refined Starch Products	0-1	
Soft Drink, Fruit Drinks	1 cup (250 ml) or less	
Other Foods High in Sugar or Saturated Fat	None or very few	

Estimating Activity Levels

Record your guess as to the number of minutes that you think your child spends in moderate activity, vigorous activity and screen time each day. Don't worry about the precise definition of moderate and vigorous activity. Just think of vigorous as meaning hard (hard to speak while doing it) and moderate as meaning easy (easy to speak while doing it). Watching television, surfing the internet and playing computer or video games make up screen time.

Activity Level Estimate		
Type of Activity	**Recommended Gold Level Daily Minutes**	**Your Guess**
Moderate Physical Activity	60 minutes	
Vigorous Physical Activity	30 minutes	
Screen Time	60 minutes maximum	

CASE STUDY Andrea's Program

Food Assessment

At Miss Nelson's suggestion, Andrea put all her lunch items out on the desk. There were four chocolate cookies, a can of pop, a peanut butter and jam sandwich on white bread, and an apple. Andrea didn't eat a lot of vegetables, although she did enjoy eating fruit. She told Miss Nelson that she ate fruit with almost every meal. "That's super!" exclaimed Miss Nelson, but also said that Andrea needed to eat more vegetables and whole grain foods.

When Miss Nelson handed her a copy of a guide for healthy eating, Andrea noticed that the number of servings allotted for things like the cookies and pop that were regularly included in her diet was very small compared to fruits, vegetables, and grains. It really got Andrea thinking; even exchanging that white bread for whole grain bread would be a healthier choice.

continued on page 245

3-Day Nutrition Diary

A 3-day nutrition diary is a record of the type and amount of food your child has eaten on 3 separate days throughout a single week. One of the 3 days must be during the weekend because food choices and selection can be different when there is less organization to the day. A 3-day nutrition diary will be kept during the assessment week and for the first 4 weeks of the program, after which it can be kept monthly.

This diary has three important purposes: it can show the potentially less healthy eating choices that a child is making; it can guide your child toward alternative healthy eating choices; and it can be used when setting goals for having better nutrition.

Grouping Foods

Calcium Sources

One serving of calcium is 300 mg, which is about the amount in a cup of milk. You may need to refer to the "Calcium Content of Common Foods" chart given in Chapter 5, "Food, Weight, and Health: Part 1" (page 136). The daily recommended calcium needed for 4- to 8-year-olds is 800 mg and for 9- to 18-year-olds it is 1300 mg.

Refined Starch Products

White breads and bread products are measured in the same way as whole-grain foods. Be sure to look at the serving sizes for the whole-grain category when determining number of servings for the Refined Starch Products category.

Potatoes

Only sweet potatoes are recorded in the vegetables group. Because they are high in starch, we would not recommend that white potatoes be eaten in the same amounts as the other vegetables. Regular white potatoes are part of the Refined Starch Products category.

Meat Alternatives

Additional servings from the Legumes, Nuts, Seeds category are counted as 'meat alternatives.' For example, if your child eats a sandwich with 1 serving of peanut butter, 1 serving of almonds for a snack, a salad with 1 serving of beans, and soup with 1 serving of tofu, your child can count these as 2 servings from Legumes, Nuts, Seeds and 2 servings from Fish, Poultry, Eggs, Lean Meat — meat alternatives.

Estimating Serving Sizes

When keeping score for the nutrition diary, you will need to find out the number of servings of foods eaten in each food category. Suppose your child ate a breakfast made up of one glass of milk, half of a whole-wheat bagel with 2 tablespoons of natural peanut butter, and a medium-sized apple. The apple counts for 1 serving in the "fruit" category, the half bagel counts for 1 serving in the "whole grains" category, the tablespoon of peanut butter counts as 1 serving in the "legumes" category, and the glass of milk counts as 1 serving in the "calcium" category. You may need to refer to the following chart often in the beginning as you are learning about correct serving sizes.

Food Group	Serving	Measure (1 cup = 250 ml)
Vegetables	Leafy vegetables	1 cup
	Raw, cooked, or canned vegetables	½ cup
Fruit	Medium-sized fruit, such as an apple, banana, orange, or pear	1 piece
	Chopped, cooked, or canned fruit	½ cup
	Dried fruit	¼ cup
Whole Grains	Thin slice of bread	50 g
	3-inch bread roll	50 g
	½ a typical size bagel	50 g
	½ a typical size pita bread	50 g
	½ of a typical muffin	50 g
	Whole-grain rice	½ cup
	Whole-grain pasta	½ cup
	Breakfast cereal	30 g
	Oatmeal	¾ cup
Legumes, Nuts, Seeds	Raw or Cooked Dry Beans	½–1 cup
	Nuts or Seeds	¼ cup
	Peanut butter	2 tbsp
	Legumes	½–1 cup
	Tofu	⅓ cup (100 grams)
Fish, Poultry, Eggs, Lean Meat	Fish, Poultry, Lean Meat	2-3 ounces (50-100 grams)
	Eggs	1–2
Calcium Sources	Non-dairy source	300 mg
	Milk	1 cup
	Cheese	50 grams (3"x1"x1")
	Yogurt	¾ cup
	Cottage Cheese	1 cup
	Processed Cheese	2 slices
	Frozen Yogurt, Pudding, Low-fat ice-cream	½ cup
		½ cup
Refined Starch Products	Cooked rice	½ cup
	Cooked pasta	½ cup
	Mashed potatoes	½ cup
	Baked potato	1 small
Soft Drinks, Fruit Drinks	Any	½ cup

3-Day Nutrition Diary

Now you are ready to complete the 3-day nutrition diary log and score card. In many cases, it is most useful to write in this nutrition diary at the end of each of the 3 days you are keeping track. Choose which 3 days your will keep track of in advance so that you and your child don't forget. You may find that the best way to help your child remember all of the foods they ate during the day is to divide the day up and ask them about specific meals and snacks.

Instructions

1. Record the food items your child eats at each meal and snack over a 3-day period.
2. Put each of the food items eaten into one of the listed food groups.
3. Estimate the serving or portion size for each food eaten.
4. Make copies of this form for setting weekly goals and recording weekly successes during the first few weeks of the program.

Other Sugar and Saturated Fat Foods

Under this food group include other processed foods that are high in saturated fat, sugar, or both. There are no specific serving sizes set for these 'other' foods. Instead, record the number of these foods that are eaten each day. The goal is to keep these foods to a minimum because they are the most common source of excess energy and place your child at risk for gaining weight and for suffering health problems.

For example, foods in this category would include the following:

☐ Cakes, cookies, crackers and candy

☐ High-fat meat (white fat visible), such as deli meats and chicken with skin. You may want to look at the list of high fat meats given in Chapter 5, "Food, Weight, and Health: Part 1" (page 132).

☐ High-fat dairy products (including butter) and margarine. You may want to look at the list of dairy products given in Chapter 5, "Food, Weight, and Health: Part 1" (page 138).

Nutrition Log: Week 1					
Meal	**Week Day 1**	**Servings**	**Week Day 2**	**Servings**	**Weekend Day 3**	**Servings**
Example: Breakfast Fruit	1 apple	1	1 orange	1	None	0
Breakfast						
Vegetable						
Fruit						
Whole Grains						
Legumes, Nuts and Seeds						
Fish, Poultry, Eggs, Lean Meat						
Calcium Sources (Dairy/Non-Dairy)						
Refined Starch Products						
Soft Drinks, Fruit Drinks						
Other Sugar and Saturated Fat Foods		Number:		Number:		Number:
Lunch						
Vegetable						
Fruit						
Whole Grains						
Nuts, Legumes						
Fish, Poultry, Eggs, Lean Meat						
Calcium (Dairy/Vegetables)						
Refined Starches						
Soft Drinks, Fruit Drinks						
Other Sugar and Saturated Fat Foods		Number:		Number:		Number:

Nutrition Log: Week 1 (cont.)						
Meal	**Week Day 1**	**Servings**	**Week Day 2**	**Servings**	**Weekend Day 3**	**Servings**
Dinner						
Vegetable						
Fruit						
Whole Grains						
Legumes, Nuts, Seeds						
Fish, Poultry, Eggs, Lean Meat						
Calcium Sources (Dairy/Non-Dairy)						
Refined Starch Products						
Soft Drinks, Fruit Drinks						
Other Sugar and Saturated Fat Foods		Number:		Number:		Number:
Snacks						
Vegetable						
Fruit						
Whole Grains						
Legumes, Nuts, and Seeds						
Fish, Poultry, Eggs, Lean Meat						
Calcium Sources (Dairy/Non-Dairy)						
Refined Starch Products						
Soft Drinks, Fruit Drinks						
Other Sugar and Saturated Fat Foods		Number:		Number:		Number:

Average Daily Servings

Now you can calculate the average number of servings per day in each food group for a typical week.

Instructions

1. Add the total number of servings for each food group eaten over all 3 days.
2. Divide that number by 3 to determine the average number of servings eaten per day for each food group.
3. Record these average numbers on the scorecard that follows.
4. Make several copies of this form for setting weekly goals and recording weekly successes during the first few weeks of the program.

Average Daily Servings: Week 1		
Food Group	**Total Servings Eaten Over 3 Days**	**Average Daily Servings**
Vegetable		
Fruit		
Whole Grains		
Legumes, Nuts, and Seeds		
Fish, Poultry, Eggs, Lean Meat		
Calcium Sources (Dairy/Non-Dairy)		
Refined Starch Products		
Soft Drinks, Fruit Drinks		
Other Sugar and Saturated Fat Foods	Number:	Number:

3-Day Nutrition Diary Scorecard

After you have recorded the types and amounts of food your child has eaten during an average day, the healthiness of an average day's nutrition can be determined by comparing the average numbers on scorecard to the gold level numbers for nutrition.

Instructions

1. Check off the number of servings of each food group eaten on the average day. One symbol on the nutrition scorecard always represents 1 serving, or 1 product for 'other' foods.
2. Then check off the "start level" for the average day — copper, bronze, silver, gold, or 'red' flag. For example, check off the number of boxes corresponding to the number of servings to determine the program level. So, if your child had 2 servings of vegetables, you should be checking off copper.
3. Finally, compare the "start level" with the "program level" column to see the healthy weight final nutrition goal for your child. As the program advances week-by-week, you will set higher goals, such as from moving from copper to bronze level in the first week.
4. Make several copies of this form for setting weekly goals and recording weekly achievements during the first few weeks of the program.

Wholesome Versus Processed Food Groups

The scorecard divides food groups into "wholesome" and "processed." Your child should aim to replace processed foods with wholesome foods as the program progresses.

Program levels are shown for particular numbers of servings in each category of the Wholesome Foods section. By looking over the nutrition diary and counting the number of servings eaten from each category, parents and children can find out what program level has been accomplished. For example, if a child had three servings of fruit over the course of the whole day, then the gold level for the fruit category would be accomplished for that day.

Program levels are also shown for particular numbers of servings in each category of the Processed Foods section. Keeping the number and size of servings lower is healthier. The scorecard starts at the gold level in each category and is lowered as they eat more and more processed food. For example, if they had two servings of processed starches, they would be at the silver level for the Refined Starch Products category.

Red Flag Warnings

The "red' flag warns that your child has exceeded the maximum recommended number of servings in the category. Being at the red flag level increases the likelihood of weight gain and health problems. Your child should make it a priority to always stay below the red flag level.

Start Level

The start level for each food group provides a yardstick to assess your child's eating habits at the start of the program and to plot your child's progress week by week during the program.

Gold Level

Over the course of the program, your child's aim is to achieve the gold level in each of the food categories on almost all days of the week — and to maintain the gold level for the rest of their life.

Nutrition Scorecard: Week 1			
Food Group	**Servings**	**Start Level**	**Program Level**
Wholesome Foods			
Vegetables	□ □ □ □ □ □ □	□ Copper □ Bronze □ Silver □ Gold	Copper: 1-2 Bronze: 3-4 Silver: 5 **Gold: 6+**
Fruit	□ □ □	□ Copper □ Bronze □ Silver □ Gold	Copper: 0 Bronze: 1 Silver: 2 **Gold: 3**
Whole Grains	□ □ □ □ □ □	□ Copper □ Bronze □ Silver □ Gold	Copper: 1-2 Bronze: 3 Silver: 4 **Gold: 5+**
Legumes, Nuts, Seeds	□ □ □	□ Copper □ Bronze □ Silver □ Gold	Copper: 0 Bronze: 1 Silver: 2 **Gold: 3**
Fish, Poultry, Eggs, Lean Meat	□ □ □	□ Copper □ Bronze □ Silver □ Gold	Copper: 0 Bronze: 1 Silver: 1-2 **Gold: 2-3**

Nutrition Scorecard: Week 1 (cont.)

Food Group	Servings	Start Level	Program Level
Wholesome Foods			
Calcium Sources	⚐ ☐ ☐ ☐	☐ Red Flag ☐ Copper ☐ Bronze ☐ Silver ☐ Gold	Red Flag: 0 Copper: 1 Bronze: 2 Silver: 3 **Gold: 4**
Processed Foods			
Refined Starch Products	☐ ☐ ☐ ☐ ☐ ⚐	☐ Gold ☐ Silver ☐ Bronze ☐ Copper ☐ Red Flag	**Gold: 0-1** Silver: 2 Bronze: 3 Copper: 4 Red Flag: 5+
Soft Drinks, Fruit Drinks	☐ ☐ ☐ ☐ ⚐	☐ Gold ☐ Silver ☐ Bronze ☐ Copper ☐ Red Flag	**Gold: 0-1** Silver: 2 Bronze: 3 Copper: 4 Red Flag: 5+
Other Sugar and Saturated Fat Foods	Total number of "other" foods: ☐ ☐ ☐ ☐ ☐ ⚐	☐ Gold ☐ Silver ☐ Bronze ☐ Copper ☐ Red Flag	**Gold: 0** Silver: 1-2 Bronze: 3-4 Copper: 5-6 Red Flag: 6+

Q: **What if we can't be exact with our serving size or numbers?**

A: It is almost impossible to know the exact amounts of food your child is eating in both the wholesome and processed food categories. They will have to rely on their memory quite a bit and they'll simply have to make their best guesses. The important thing is not to guess lower on the processed food categories and higher on the more nutritious food. Encourage your children to be honest about what they are eating and how much. Let them know they will not be punished or criticized. The reason for keeping track is so that children can learn about their eating habits and see general improvements as they go through the program. Once your child is eating more nutritious food more often and has become more physically active, they will be healthier and get to a healthier body weight.

Drinks and Juices

100% Pure Fruit Juice

If your child drinks juices, we recommend that you buy pure fruit juice, not fruit drinks. However, even pure juice can be a source of excessive calories so moderation is the key. Notice that if young people drink 1 cup (250 ml) of pure fruit juice, they still meet the gold level for this category. More than this amount is not recommended. It is actually better for the child to eat a piece of fruit than to just drink the fruit's juice.

Soft Drinks

Even though drinking 1 cup (250 ml) of soft drinks would still keep your child at the gold level in this category, there are really no nutritional benefits to these drinks. Slowly decreasing their soft drink intake to 'none' or, at most, 'only on special occasions' is recommended. Remember, most soft drinks are sold in servings much longer than 1 cup.

'Diet' Soft Drinks

Artificially sweetened drinks (diet soft drinks and those 'sweetened' with aspartame or sucralose, for example) do not count as drinks in this section. However, we do encourage drinking water instead of any of these drinks. Diet soft drinks may still increase the chances of tooth decay because of their acidity, and many of them have caffeine.

CASE STUDY Andrea's Program

Activity Assessment

Miss Nelson asked Andrea to think about what kinds of physical activity she did. Besides her one trip to dance class, the only physical activity Andrea participated in was gym class at school and that wasn't even every day. After school she usually watched a couple hours of television. After dinner she chatted with her friends with an instant message program on her computer.

Andrea knew from her experience at dance class that she wasn't doing enough physical activity. "I don't like sports, though," Andrea told Miss Nelson, while envisioning falling on her face trying to play basketball. Miss Nelson assured Andrea that physical activity was more than just playing sports, and that it would be easy for her to increase her activity levels by 30 minutes per day, while decreasing the time she spent doing things like watching TV or chatting on the computer.

continued on page 256

3-Day Activity Diary

A 3-day activity diary is a record of your child's activity or inactivity during 3 separate days throughout a single week. One of the 3 days must be during the weekend because activity choices can be quite different on days when your child is not in school.

Like the 3-day nutrition diary, the 3-day activity diary has three important purposes: it can help your child become aware of their level of inactivity; it can help guide you and your child toward meaningful amounts of physical activity; and it can be used when setting goals for increasing activity and decreasing inactivity.

A 3-day activity diary will be kept during the beginning assessment week of the program and for the following 3 weeks, after which it can be kept monthly.

3-Day Activity Diary Log

You may find that the best way to help your child remember all of the activities they took part in during the day is to ask about each specific time during that day.

Instructions

1. Record the type of activity (including "screen time") and the time spent for each activity.
2. Check off the level of activity — screen time, moderate, or vigorous.
3. Make several copies of this form for setting weekly goals and recording weekly successes during the first few weeks of the program.
4. As the program progresses week-by-week, you will set higher goals, such as moving from copper to bronze level, in the second week.

Activity Log: Week 1					
Time of Day	**Activity Description**	**Time Spent in Minutes**	**Moderate**	**Vigorous**	**Screen Time**
Weekday 1 Date:					
Example 7:00 a.m.	Jogging	20 minutes	✔		
Weekday 2 Date:					
Weekend Day 3 Date:					

Average Daily Activities

Now you can now calculate the average activities per day in a typical week for each level of activity.

Instructions

1. Add the number of minutes for each level of activity — moderate, vigorous, and screen time.
2. Divide by 3 to determine the average daily time spent in minutes for each level of activity.
3. Record these average numbers on the scorecard that follows.
4. Make several copies of this form for setting weekly goals and recording weekly successes during the first few weeks of the program.

Average Daily Activities: Week 1		
Level of Activity	**Total Minutes for 3 Days**	**Average Daily Minutes**
Moderate		
Vigorous		
Screen Time		

3-Day Activity Diary Scorecard

After you have calculated the levels and average time spent for your child's activity during the average day, the current level of the day's activities can be determined using a score-card and compared to the program levels for activity.

Instructions

1. Check off the number of minutes of activity at each level — moderate, vigorous, and screen time.
2. Then check off the "start level" on the average day — first steps, copper, bronze, silver, gold, or 'red' flag. For example, check off the box that corresponds to the amount of minutes spent in each activity and then determine the program level. So, if your child spent 25 minutes in moderate activity, you should be checking off Copper.
3. Finally, compare the "start level" with the "program level" column to see the healthy weight activity goal for your child.
4. Make several copies of this form for setting weekly goals and recording weekly successes during the first few weeks of the program.

Activity Scorecard: Week 1			
Type of Activity	**Time Spent per Average Day** (Duration in Minutes)	**Start Level**	**Program Level** (minutes per day)
Moderate	0-20 21-30 31-40 41-50 51-60 ☐ ☐ ☐ ☐ ☐	☐ First Steps ☐ Copper ☐ Bronze ☐ Silver ☐ Gold	First Steps: 0–20 Copper: 21-30 Bronze: 31-40 Silver: 41-50 **Gold: 60+**
Vigorous	0-10 11-15 16-20 21-25 26-30 ☐ ☐ ☐ ☐ ☐	☐ First Steps ☐ Copper ☐ Bronze ☐ Silver ☐ Gold	First Steps: 0–10 Copper: 11-15 Bronze: 16-20 Silver: 21-25 **Gold: 30+**
Screen Time	>150 120 90 < 60 (1 hr) ☐ ☐ ☐ ☐	☐ Gold ☐ Silver ☐ Bronze ☐ Copper ☐ Red Flag	**Gold: <60** Silver: 61-90 Bronze: 91-120 Copper: 121-150 Red Flag: >150

Moderate and Vigorous Physical Activity

To determine if the activity is moderate or vigorous, you can look at the "MET Charts for Moderate and Vigorous Activities" for a list of the most common moderate and vigorous level activities, ordered by their MET value.

The MET value for a particular activity shows how much more energy our body uses compared to when we are sitting still. The higher the MET value of an activity, the more energy the body uses in doing that activity. We group any activities that have MET values between 3 and 6 as moderate physical activity. Vigorous activities are those that have a MET value of more than 6.

Imagine that your child walked to school today, played tetherball at recess, and then played baseball outside after school. These are all activities listed in the "Moderate Physical Activities" list. If the walk to school took 15 minutes, the tetherball game lasted 10 minutes, and the baseball game lasted 30 minutes, your child will have done 55 minutes of moderate activity for the day. Looking at the activity scorecard, your child would be at the gold level for moderate activity.

Screen Time

Screen time is the total amount of time spent watching television, playing video games, and playing games on the computer (including surfing the internet for fun) during the day.

School-related computer use for homework is not counted as screen time.

Start Level

The start level for each activity type provides a yardstick to assess your child's activity habits at the start of the program and to assess your child's progress week by week during the program.

Gold Standard

Over the course of the program, your child's aim is to get to the gold level in each activity category on most days of the week — and to maintain the gold level for the rest of their life.

> **Q:** **What if my child has taken part in an activity that is not on the list?**
>
> **A:** If your child has participated in an activity that is not in the moderate or vigorous physical activity lists we have provided, just try to find the closest match or most similar activity in the list to determine if it is a moderate or vigorous activity.

MET Moderate Activities		
Type of Activity	**Description**	**METS**
Walking	Walking leisurely	3.5
Bicycling	Bicycling leisurely	4
Dancing	Light dance: ballet or modern, twist, jazz, tap, jitterbug	4.8

MET Moderate Activities (cont.)

Type of Activity	Description	METS
Other:		
Land Activities	Trampoline	3.5
Land Activities	Gymnastics in general	4
Land Activities	Hacky-sack	4
Land Activities	Horseback riding in general	4
Land Activities	Ping-Pong	4
Land Activities	Volleyball	4
Land Activities	Badminton	4.5
Land Activities	Golf (without cart)	4.5
Land Activities	Hopscotch, dodge ball, playground, t-ball, tetherball, race-type games	5
Land Activities	Skateboarding	5
Land Activities	Softball or baseball (recreational)	5
Land Activities	Basketball (recreational)	6
Land Activities	Boxing, punching bag	6
Land Activities	Paddleball	6
Water Activities	Sailing	3
Water Activities	Canoeing (leisurely)	4
Water Activities	Kayaking	5
Water Activities	Snorkeling	5
Water Activities	Waterskiing	6
Winter Activities	Downhill skiing (leisurely)	6
Music Activities	Playing the drums	4
Home Activities	Sweeping garage, sidewalk, or outside of house	4
Home Activities	Raking lawn	4.3
Home Activities	Clearing land, hauling branches, wheelbarrow chores	5
Home Activities	Digging, spading, filling garden, composting	5
Home Activities	Mowing lawn (push mower)	5.5
Home Activities	Snow shoveling	6

MET Vigorous Activities		
Type of Activity	**Description**	**METS**
Running	Jogging and running	7
Bicycling	Bicycling (moderate effort)	8
Dancing	Aerobic classes, hip-hop (moderate effort)	6.5
Other:		
Land Activities	Racquet ball	7
Land Activities	Roller-skating	7
Land Activities	Soccer	7
Land Activities	Tennis	7
Land Activities	Basketball (competitive game)	8
Land Activities	Football	8
Land Activities	Ultimate frisbee	8
Land Activities	Field hockey	8
Land Activities	Lacrosse	8
Land Activities	Skipping rope	8
Land Activities	Boxing, sparring	9
Land Activities	Martial arts: judo, jujitsu, karate, kick boxing, taekwando	10
Land Activities	Rugby	10
Land Activities	Rock climbing	11
Land Activities	Handball	12
Land Activities	Squash	12
Land Activities	Rollerblading	12
Water Activities	Canoeing, rowing (moderate effort)	7
Water Activities	Swimming laps	7
Winter Activities	Ice skating	7
Winter Activities	Cross-country skiing (leisurely)	7
Winter Activities	Ice hockey	8
Winter Activities	Downhill skiing (moderate effort)	8
Winter Activities	Snowshoeing	8

Progressive Activity

Steady improvement over several weeks and months is the aim of physical activity. Try not to achieve a gold level in 1 week if you are now just taking first steps. The following chart shows the recommended progression for moderate and vigorous activities, based on "Canada's Physical Activity Guide to Healthy Active Living" from Health Canada.

Week	Daily Moderate Activity	Daily Vigorous Activity
Week 1-5	First Steps (20 min)	First Steps (10 min)
Week 8	Copper (30 min)	Copper (11-15 min)
Week 12	Bronze (40 min)	Bronze (16-20 min)
Week 16	Silver (50 min)	Silver (21-25 min)
Week 20	Gold (60 min or more)	Gold (30 min or more)

Height and Weight Measurement Records

As part of the assessment stage of the program, you need to record your child's current height and weight. These records should be made every two weeks so that you can check your child's height and weight over the course of the program.

You can also calculate how close your child is to their healthy weight target by using the body mass index (BMI) charts provided in Chapter 2, "How Do I Know If My Child Is Overweight" (page 61).

There are good reasons for making the measurements: the healthy weight for your child is based partly on their height, which may change with time if they are growing; if your child is gaining excessive amounts of weight than needed to match their height, this can be promptly detected; and you and your child will be able to see their progress in the program over time.

Instructions

1. Pick a day of the week (Monday, for example) for recording measurements, and use that same day every other week (biweekly) for an update. Record the date.
2. Measure your child's height and record it. Record the measurement in inches or centimeters. Use the same units of measure — metric or imperial.
3. Measure your child's weight. Record the measurement pounds or kilograms. Always use the same weigh scale.
4. Calculate your child's target weight using the body mass index (BMI) charts described in Chapter 2 (page 61).
5. Subtract your child's current weight from the target weight and record the difference. This difference then becomes the total weight loss goal.

Height, Weight, and Target Weight Chart				
Date	Height	Weight	Target Weight	Difference
Week Date:				

Stage 1 Review (Week 1)

☐ Family Nutrition and Activity Worksheet
☐ Child's Nutrition and Activity Worksheet
☐ 3-Day Nutrition Diary: Log and Scorecard
☐ 3-Day Activity Diary: Log and Scorecard
☐ Height, Weight, and Target Weight Chart

Make sure that you are comfortable with keeping and scoring the 3-day nutrition and activity diaries before you begin using them with your child. You may want to practice using them for yourself for a week. You may even discover that your own nutrition or level of physical activity could be improved.

STAGE 2

Setting Goals and Rewards (Week 2)

Now that you have completed the program assessment, you are ready to start helping your child set goals to make healthy changes.

This program depends a great deal on teaching your child practical goal-setting skills and then using these goals to make changes in their lifestyle. The program can only succeed when you and your child use practical goal setting.

Stage 2 Preview (Week 2)

☐ Goal of the Week Worksheet
☐ Goal of the Week Evaluation Questionnaire
☐ 3-Day Nutrition Diary: Log and Scorecard
☐ 3-Day Activity Diary: Log and Scorecard

Value of Setting Goals

- Just making goals will increase your child's success at whatever they attempt to do.
- Goals will help your child to accept and deal with challenges.
- When the goals are actually written down, they are even more likely to be accomplished.
- Goals will give your child a sense of control over their nutrition and physical activity.
- Goals allow your child to recognize and seek situations, places or people that help them to succeed.
- Goals allow your child to recognize and avoid situations, places or people that may hamper their success.
- Accomplishing goals will boost your child's self-confidence and how good they feel about themselves.
- Self-confidence from successfully meeting goals will help your child take on even more difficult challenges.
- Goals give your child a real sense of purpose for what they are doing.
- Setting goals gives your child a plan for getting success.

CASE STUDY Andrea's Program

Setting Family Goals

Andrea came home from school that day and told her mom all about her meeting with Miss Nelson. Andrea knew she needed to make changes in the way she ate and exercised, but she confided in her mom that she had doubts about her ability to make the necessary changes. Andrea's mom suggested that it might be easier if the whole family got involved. After all, though not everyone in her family had a goal of losing weight, there were ways in which everyone could improve their activity and eating habits. Andrea liked the idea of working together as a family.

They decided that since they rarely ate all of the healthy foods that they should in a day, a checklist would be helpful. Each family member's name was listed on the chart along with the amount of servings of different food groups that they should each eat daily. Each person tallied in each box the number of foods from each category that they consumed in a given day. This was a great idea because everyone could see which food groups they had already eaten that day, as well as what food groups they still needed to cover. Also, they had decided as a family to cut back on how often they ate out and ordered in food to once a week at most.

The family decided that they could use a similar chart for exercise. On the top of the chart the day of the week was listed where each family member could fill in the amount of time they participated in physical activities that day. As well, they decided that it would be a good idea to take family walks or jogs together in order to get more exercise as well as help bring the family closer together.

They came up with some other healthy goals, such as not taking food out of the kitchen and not eating while watching TV. Other ideas, such as walking to school or the mall as opposed to taking a car, were easy to implement. Finally, the family decided to devote at least one Sunday a month to an outing or activity that involved some exercise. One suggestion was walking around downtown for the day. Although they lived just outside of the city, they didn't get to explore it much. They would also visit the local museum and art gallery, activities which involved much walking and were also educational.

continued on page 262

Nutrition and Activity Goals

Nutrition and activity goals can be either "knowledge" or "action" goals.

- **Knowledge Goals:** Completing knowledge goals teaches your child important ideas and information about improving their nutrition and activity.
- **Action Goals:** Completing action goals involves your child actually making some changes that will improve their nutrition and activity.

Sample Program Goals

Each week your child will choose one nutrition goal and one activity goal from a list of possible program goals. Listed here are examples of some of these program goals. We have provided enough program goals to allow your child to go many months without repeating the same goal. Some of these program goals can be accomplished in 1 week, such as "Eat more fruit this week," while others may take longer, such as "Run a 3-kilometer race." The plan should be to keep all of the changes going successfully while continuing to add new ones.

Each goal should be stated in writing using the same wording: *"This week I shall:"*

Nutrition Goals: Knowledge
"This week I shall..."

Grocery Store Shopping Goals

- Help my parents do the grocery shopping. Take to the grocery store a copy of my 3-day nutrition scorecard as a guide to buying healthy food.
- Explore the fruit and vegetable section of the store and buy different colored items and foods high in calcium and high in fiber.
- Buy and eat a fruit and a vegetable that I've never tried before.
- Look for plain nuts and seeds in the bulk food section to buy for snacks. Avoid heavily salted and sugar-coated nuts and seeds.
- Add fresh or frozen fish to the grocery cart.
- Choose low-fat or fat-free milk, yogurt, and cheese by reading the labels carefully.
- Read the food labels on packaged and processed foods before buying them. Make a list of alternative fresh whole foods to eat.
- Choose fresh fruit juices or bottled water rather than sweet fruit drinks and soda or pop.
- Choose not to buy high-saturated fat and high-sugar items found in the snack food aisle of the store. Substitute with fresh fruit and plain nuts.
- Choose not to buy quick snack chocolate bars and candies stocked near the check-out counter.

Nutrition Goals

Apply the white fat rule (no or low visible white fat) when buying meat, poultry, and deli.

Apply the white grain rule (no or low white grains) when picking bread, muffins, wraps, bagels, rice, and other processed starchy foods.

Nutrition Goals

Help mom or dad cut up vegetables and prepare other healthy ingredients for meals and snacks.

Eat breakfast every day before going to school. I won't skip breakfast.

Food Planning Goals

- Plan meals and snacks with my family for the week to achieve gold levels for the various food groups.
- Tour the kitchen and pay attention to the amounts of fresh whole foods versus the processed and preserved foods in the cupboards and refrigerator. Reduce or remove unhealthy food items.
- Choose a healthy recipe from a book, newspaper or the internet to prepare. Help my parents shop for the ingredients or make a list for them.
- Serve fancy fruit, vegetables, and healthy dips at family birthday parties and other holiday celebrations.

School Food Environment Goals

- Tour the school and pay attention to the food and drink choices on the cafeteria menu and in the vending machines. Ask my teachers if healthier food items can be added to the menu or the machines.
- Eat fresh vegetables and a piece of fruit with the school food on hot dog, pizza and sub days.

Food Cravings Goals

- Make a list of all the times when I'm tempted to eat more food than I'm really hungry for. For each of these, give a solution that would help prevent me from eating as much.
- Make a list of all the times when I'm tempted to eat sweets or higher-fat foods. For each, give an alternative food I could choose to eat instead or an activity that would distract me from thinking about these types of food.

Nutrition Goals: Action
"This week I shall..."

Breakfast Goals

- Eat a breakfast that includes fruit, a protein source (such as peanut butter, cheese, or milk), and a carbohydrate source (whole-wheat bread or bagel, whole-grain cereal, oatmeal).
- Prepare what to eat for breakfast the night before so that if there isn't a lot of time in the morning, I can still have breakfast.
- Eat a piece of fruit with breakfast instead of having a fruit drink or fruit juice. Drink low-fat milk or water instead.
- Add fresh or frozen fruit to whole grain breakfast cereals to make them taste better without using sugar.

Lunch Goals

- Prepare a healthy lunch at home to take to school instead of buying lunch at school. Include one or more servings of vegetables.
- Choose not to eat deli meats with visible white fat.
- Choose not to eat lunch convenience foods, such as high-sugar granola bars, fruit drink boxes and cans of soda/pop.
- Choose whole-grain bread for a sandwich, whole wheat bagels or whole wheat wraps.
- Choose not to eat convenience and fast-foods served in the cafeteria and sold from vending machines.

Snack Goals

- Bring fruit, cut-up vegetables, or nuts to school for a snack. Eat some of these for after-school snacks.
- Not eat food while watching TV or sitting at the computer.

Dinner Goals

- Try eating cut up vegetables with a low-fat, low-calorie dip with dinner.
- Add fresh or frozen fruit to salads.
- Help mom and dad prepare lean meats with little or no white fat visible and poultry without the skin for entrées.
- Choose lower-fat or fat-free milk, yogurt, and cheese.
- Choose fruit as a dessert after dinner instead of baked goods or sweet puddings.
- Ask my parents to add fresh or frozen fruit to home-baked goods.

Eating Out Goals

- Avoid the high-fat, high-sugar and high-salt salad dressings and sauces used for salads and dips.
- Find take-out restaurants that serve healthier foods that are not deep-fried and that offer a variety of vegetables and even fruit.

Drink and Beverage Goals

- Reduce the number of sodas/pop consumed.
- Reduce the amount of fruit juice or fruit drinks consumed per sitting by 50% or more.
- Replace sodas/pop and fruit drinks/fruit juice with water.
- Remove soda/pop and fruit drinks/fruit juice from the house and serve them only as special treats outside the home.

Nutrition Goals

Prepare a high-fiber salad, including several vegetables, to eat before the dinner entrée.

Choose healthy food alternatives from the menu at fast-food restaurants.

Family Food Habit Goals

- Help choose particular days when the whole family will eat together.
- Try to set a regular mealtime for dinner and stick to it.
- Only eat food in the kitchen or dining room.
- Try using the plate model for portions: 2 to 3 parts of the plate is covered by vegetables (ideally fresh not canned), 1 part by a whole-grain starchy food (brown rice or whole grain pastas, for example), and 1 part quarter by a low-fat protein source (lean meat, fish, eggs, or beans, for example).

Activity Goals: Knowledge
"This week I shall…"

Fitness Goals

> **Activity Goals**
>
> Test out a school or community sports program at a level that seems to fit.
>
> Ask friends what activities they are involved with and see if any of those activities seem interesting. Ask them to introduce me to their coaches and teammates.

- Explore with my parents the parks, sports fields, arenas, and other recreation centers in the community to see what they have to offer for play and sports activities.
- Use park playsets, baseball diamonds, and hockey rinks for fun activities with friends and family.
- Look into the gym, fitness, and sports programs offered at school as intramural and varsity activities.
- Choose a weekend or a day after school to look into all the different sports teams active in the community.
- Take swimming, martial arts, sailing, horseback riding, or dance lessons or some other form of activity lessons.

Exercise Goals

- Tour a local health club or gym to see what aerobic endurance activities are offered for young people and what equipment can be used for strength and flexibility activities.
- Find out if there are any classes offered especially for young people like me.
- Visit an exercise equipment store with my parents and discover if there is any equipment I would like to use, such as exercise balls, exercise bands, and exercise videos.

Home Activity Goals

- Do a survey and write down all the ways that I can think of being more active inside the home and outside in the yard.

Activity Goals: Action
"This week I shall..."

Daily Living Activity Goals
- Help mom or dad clear the table, wash the dishes, and clean up the kitchen.
- Walk to school.
- Walk the dog.
- Walk up the stairs instead of using the escalator or elevator.
- Clean up my own room and help clean up the house.
- Help shovel the snow, mow the lawn, or rake the leaves.
- Play with friends — tag, catch, basketball, soccer, ball hockey — as a group.

Moderate Activity Goals
- Go for a brisk walk around the block after school or after dinner.
- Walk up hills or climb stairs.
- Spend ½ hour playing in the water and swimming at the community pool.

Endurance Activity Goals
- Go on a walk and then run for 1 minute after every 10 minutes of walking.
- Go on a walk and then run for 2 minutes after every 10 minutes of walking.
- Go on a 5-minute bike ride after school or on weekends.
- Go on a 10-minute bike ride after school or on weekends.
- Spend 15 minutes swimming laps at the pool.
- Run an organized 5-km race.

Strength and Flexibility Activity Goals
- Ask my phys-ed instructor at school for strength-training and stretching routines suited to my level of fitness.
- Practice basic stretching activities — touching toes, knee bends, resistance training.

Screen Activity Goals
- Reduce television and computer game time activity to 1 to 2 hours per day.
- Remove the television from the kitchen, dining room, and bedrooms.

Nutrition Goals

Replace one hour of television watching with an hour spent playing outside in the yard or at the park.

CASE STUDY Andrea's Program

Personalized Goals

Andrea decided to set some personal goals that she wanted to reach. She didn't want to look only at weight as the criterion for how healthy she was. She came up with additional goals, such as being able to walk around the block in her neighborhood in a given amount of time without getting winded. She also hoped to be able to get through an entire dance class without feeling like she was going to collapse. She did set a rough goal of a weight she wanted to reach, but knew that it wasn't written in stone. After all, her main goal was to be healthier. She hoped to set realistic goals that were attainable, but also ones that were a bit of a challenge.

In her health class, she recalled a system that her teacher, Miss Nelson, had taught about making health-related goals. It was called the SMART way. S stood for specific, M was for measurable, A for attainable, R for realistic, and finally T for time-oriented. She tried to make her goals fit this acronym. It was a great way to check and see if her goals were written in a way so that she couldn't cheat or find loopholes that could hinder her progress.

The charts in the kitchen helped her to monitor the kinds and numbers of different foods that she ate as she tried to slowly improve her eating. She made it a goal to do some sort of physical activity at least 4 days a week for a minimum of an hour. She figured this was reasonable. She took things slowly and improved each week by aiming to add a few more minutes of physical activity to her routine and by replacing a not-so-healthy snack with a healthier choice, such as a fruit or vegetable. Lastly, she tried to get up earlier each day so that she would have enough time to be able to walk to school.

continue on page 272

Personalizing Program Goals

The program goals your child chooses also need to be personalized so that they can be accomplished more readily and more meaningfully. For example, the program goal "Eat more fruit this week" doesn't tell your child how much more, what types of fruit, or when. It doesn't identify any barriers to achieving this goal or any special family help that may be required. Your child will need to create their own specific personalized goals that accomplish the program goals they choose.

Making Better Personal Goal Statements

When putting down program goals, try to be as specific and detailed as possible. The following are some examples of both vague and more successful program goals.

Vague Program Goals	Successful Program Goals
Eat better this week	Eat more fruit this week
Run farther or faster	Run a 5-km race without stopping
Improve my health	Find out what team sports I can take part in after school
Lose excess body weight	Drink fewer cans of soda/pop this week
Get stronger	Do strength-building exercises this week

The following list shows how to change some unsuccessful personalized goals into clearer, more specific, measurable and realistic alternatives.

Successful Personalized Goals		
Program Goals	Unsuccessful Personalized Goals	More Specific and Successful Alternatives
Eat more fruit this week	I will eat one piece of fruit each day	I will eat one apple on Monday, Wednesday, and Friday with breakfast (8:00 a.m.)
Run a 3-km race without stopping	I will run after school each day of the week	I will run for 5 minutes after school (4:00 p.m.) on Monday, Tuesday, Thursday, and Friday
Watch less television this week	I will not watch as much television after school	I will go play with friends outside for 1 hour after school (4:00 p.m.) on Monday, Wednesday, and Friday instead of watching television at these times.
Eat healthy at a fast-food restaurant	The next time I am at a fast food restaurant, I'll order something healthy	I will go to a fast-food restaurant for dinner with my family on Wednesday at 6:00 p.m. I will order a grilled chicken sandwich, a salad with dressing on the side, and water.

Features of Successful Personalized Goals

When making personalized or custom-made program goals, try using the SMART way for stating personalized goals:

S: Specific: The goal is specific if you can answer exactly when, where, what, who, and how.

M: Measurable: There is an exact way to determine if goal has been accomplished.

A: Attainable: The goal is something that is actually possible to accomplish.

R: Realistic: It is very likely that the goal will be accomplished.

T: Time-oriented: It can be accomplished in a reasonable amount of time. Make adjustments for barriers that may arise.

Customize

Occasionally, your child will customize one of the program goals we have provided to make it realistic and doable for them. For example, a program goal might be to "Run an organized 5-kilometer race." Your child may decide that a 3-km race is a more realistic program goal for them to start with. After accomplishing the 3-kilometer race they may decide to customize it further to be a 10-kilometer race.

Be Creative

Your child may come up with an entirely new goal that we haven't included. That is great as long as the goal helps improve some aspect of their nutrition or physical activity. Remember, the purpose of all program goals is to bring your child to higher and higher program levels.

Goal of the Week

Accomplishing personalized goals that achieve program goals is important for the success of the program and will make sure that your child develops a healthy lifestyle. To help guide your child in making successful personalized goals, a goal of the week worksheet is useful. The goal of the week worksheet is divided into several sections. Each section asks you and your child to name the important features that will make their personalized goal successful.

Goal of the Week Worksheet

General Instructions

1. Set two personalized program goals per week and complete a goal of the week worksheet for each goal.
2. Make at least two copies of the worksheet for each week or simply copy out the sections of the worksheet each week and record the answers on a separate piece of paper.
3. Keep the goal of the week worksheets placed in a well-known location where they can be seen often so that they act as a constant reminder.
4. For more guidance in completing this worksheet, see the specific instructions that follow the worksheet.

Specific Instructions

By thoughtfully working through each section of the worksheet, your child will end up with an effective personal goal that they are likely to accomplish. You may need to review these instructions for completing the worksheet many times in the beginning stages of the program to be sure your child is properly setting goals. Initially, you may need to help your child quite a bit as they complete the form. As you and your child become more skilled at setting goals, this will be easier and take much less time.

1. What is the week in the program and the date?
Record the week number of the program and the starting date of the week. The week number and date are recorded so that, over time, you and your child will be able to look back at the goals and learn what made them successful or not. With this knowledge, your child will get better at setting personal goals that they are more likely to achieve.

2. What is the type of goal for the week?
On each goal sheet, circle the type of goal (nutrition/activity). We recommend choosing at least one personalized nutrition goal and one personalized activity goal each week. We also suggest making one a knowledge goal and one an action goal.

3. What is the specific personalized goal for the week?
Now that your child has a reason for setting a specific personalized goal for the week, they need to write it down. The goal must be written down, not just said aloud.

Goal of the Week Worksheet

1. What is the week in the program and the date?

☐ Week _____

☐ Date _____

2. What is the type of goal for the week?

☐ Nutrition   or   ☐ Activity

☐ Knowledge   or   ☐ Action

3. What is the specific personalized goal for the week?

4. What are the specific days and times for achieving the goal?

Days: Monday   Tuesday   Wednesday   Thursday   Friday   Saturday   Sunday

Times: _____   _____   _____   _____   _____   _____   _____

5. How will you keep track?

6. What preparation is needed?

7. What will help you achieve the goal?

8. What barriers might you come across and what is the plan for overcoming them?

☐ Obstacle: ☐ Obstacle:

☐ Solution: ☐ Solution:

9. Who is responsible for seeing if the goal is successfully met?

10. Is there a reward for accomplishing this goal?

4. What are the specific days and times for achieving the goal?
Specify the days and times for achieving the personalized program goal. Some goals may only need to be done once during the week and at one time, such as "I will go to the local community center on Wednesday at 4:00 p.m. and choose a group activity to become involved with." Other goals may happen three times a week or more, such as "On Monday, Wednesday, and Friday, I will eat one apple or banana with breakfast." The more specific the goal is, the more likely it will be accomplished.

5. How will you keep track?
Determine how progress toward the goal will be measured. For example, if the goal is to eat two pieces of fruit on Monday, Wednesday, and Friday at breakfast (8:00 a.m.) and lunch (12:00 p.m.), you need to record the accomplishment of that goal for the specified days. In cases like this, your child may decide to simply record it on the worksheet as a "success" for the day. No matter what the goal is, they need to use a consistent way to record it.

6. What preparation is needed? List any preparation required to begin the process of achieving the goal.

7. What will help you achieve the goal?
This is where your child can write down anything that they feel will increase the likelihood of accomplishing their goals. These can be people, places, or things … anything that helps them succeed. Some examples include having a specific friend do the goal with them, having a parent participate, getting encouragement from family and friends, going to a local park to achieve the goal instead of just staying on the street. As your child learns to discover these positive influences, they can seek them out and increase their successes.

8. What barriers might you come across and what is the plan for overcoming them?
List the factors that might make their goal more difficult to achieve. These factors may be people, places or things. For each barrier your child recognizes, help to provide creative solutions or a plan for overcoming them. Sometimes while you and your child begin to fill in this part of the worksheet, you'll discover that slightly changing the specific goal will avoid all the barriers. Other times, you and your child may

not know all of the barriers in advance. As your child attempts more and more of the goals they set, they will start to learn which barriers they commonly face and they'll be able to learn ways of avoiding or dealing with them. You can also use this question as a test of their personalized goal. If the barriers that might be faced have no solutions, the goal may not be a successful one. Be sure to make out what are barriers and what are actually excuses.

9. Who is responsible for seeing if the goal is successfully met?
Decide who will check that the goal has been completed. Most often you will be that person, but sometimes it may be a teacher or a coach or another family member. Whoever it is, your child should expect that the person will be checking up to see that they are having success with their goal and that has been completed, and maybe to offer help or encouragement. Alternatively, it will be your child's responsibility to let that person know that they have completed it.

10. Is there a reward for accomplishing this goal?
Set up ways to give positive feedback and praise for all attempted goals. Sometimes your child will set and achieve a goal that deserves some extra special attention. Maybe they've been running farther and farther over several weeks to meet their goal of running their first 5-kilometer race. Perhaps you decided that a new basketball net was the reward for finishing the race. When rewards are used properly, they are a powerful way to encourage anyone to change their behavior. Use the rewards section of the worksheet to write down any specific rewards you have determined for that goal.

Q: What happens if the goal cannot be completed as planned?

A: Weekly goals are set at the beginning of the week. Sometimes, for reasons beyond your child's control, the day or time of day set for a goal is no longer appropriate. In this case, your child can make up for it on another day. If this is not possible, your child can simply set the same goal again for the next week. Your child should not set a goal that they won't accomplish. Setting unrealistic goals will only hurt your child's self-esteem when they don't achieve them.

Preparing to Achieve Personalized Program Goals

Personalized Specific Program Goals	Preparation Needed
I will eat one apple on Monday, Wednesday, and Friday with breakfast (8:00 a.m.).	Mom needs to buy enough apples for the week.
I will run for 5 minutes after school (4:00 p.m.) on Monday, Tuesday, Thursday, and Friday	I need to get shoes that fit well and are appropriate for running. I need to make sure I have a watch to keep track of time.
I will go play with friends outside for 1 hour after school (4:00 p.m.) on Monday, Wednesday, and Friday instead of watching television at these times.	I need to arrange with my friends that I will play with them outside after school.
I will go to a fast-food restaurant for dinner with my family on Wednesday at 6:00 p.m. I will order a grilled chicken sandwich, a salad with dressing on the side, and water.	The whole family has to be told that we are going out for dinner on Wednesday. I have to make sure there aren't any other commitments that might get in the way.

Factors Helping Achievement of Personalized Program Goals

Personalized Specific Goals	Helping Factors
I will eat one apple on Monday, Wednesday, and Friday with breakfast (8:00 a.m.).	Fresh fruit is always visible on the counter. Mom will leave a note reminding me to eat fruit.
I will run for 5 minutes after school (4:00 p.m.) on Monday, Tuesday, Thursday, and Friday.	My dad will run with me on some days. My friend has agreed to run with me.
I will go play with friends outside for 1 hour after school (4:00 p.m.) on Monday, Wednesday, and Friday instead of watching television.	There is no television in my room. There is a rule: No television watching until after dinner.
I will go to a fast food restaurant for dinner with my family on Wednesday at 6:00 p.m. I will order a grilled chicken sandwich, a salad with dressing on the side, and water.	The whole family will eat healthy at a fast-food restaurant. My best friend will come with us and also try to eat healthy at a fast-food restaurant.

Barriers or Excuses Holding Back Achievements of Personalized Program Goals

Personalized Goal: I will eat one apple on Monday, Wednesday, and Friday with breakfast (8:00 a.m.)

Barrier/Excuse: I have little time in the morning to eat fruit.

Solution: Your child could prepare fruit to eat the night before or take an apple, orange, banana, or pear as they leave the house in the morning. Having too little time for fruit in the morning is more of an excuse than an barrier.

Excuse/Barrier: My sister doesn't eat fruit. She eats "junk cereal" for breakfast.

Solution: Eating fruit is healthy for everyone; your daughter should also be eating fruit at breakfast. Keeping less sugary cereal in the house will decrease temptations that make it more difficult for your child to eat more healthily.

Personalized Goal: I will run for 5 minutes after school (4:00 p.m.) on Monday, Tuesday, Thursday, and Friday.

Barriers: I don't have time to run after school because I have too much homework to do.

Solution: Allowing your child to do physical activity after school, especially after sitting all day, will improve their ability to concentrate and complete their homework. By building routine physical activity into their day, your child will become more well-organized at other times when they are completing their homework.

Personalized Goal: I will go play with friends outside for 1 hour after school (4:00 p.m.) on Monday, Wednesday, and Friday instead of watching television at these times.

Barriers: It's hard for me to avoid television when I know my sister is watching it after school.

Solution: Set a rule for the whole family that the television is only for after dinner.

Excuse: My favorite television show is on at 4:00 p.m.

Solution: Maybe the television program can be recorded and watched later on that day or another day. Your child could find an alternative to television during times when they normally watch even though they don't particularly enjoy the program.

Personalized Goal: I will go to a fast-food restaurant for dinner with my family on Wednesday at 6:00 p.m. I will order a grilled chicken sandwich, a salad with dressing on the side, and water.

Barriers: Mom may have to work late Wednesday.

Solution: Have a backup plan (another day that might be available).

Making a Deal

Sometimes you will also want to make a contract with your child to work on achieving specific goals, something you might draft for both of you to sign. This is an 'adult' thing to do and gives your child a sense of control and responsibility. The contract may also specify rewards for success. Be sure the terms are agreed upon by both parties and that the terms are then applied consistently and fairly and firmly.

Goal of the Week Evaluation

After a goal of the week has been attempted, discuss with your child if you think the goal was realistic. If the goal was realistic, it should have been successfully completed. If it wasn't completed, your child may need more practice setting more goals. Your child can use this review of previous goals when making new goals so that they will make them even more successful.

Every time a goal of the week is attempted, you should help your child complete an evaluation worksheet. Be sure to right down the answers to these questions to serve as a record when planning next week's goal of the week.

Goal of the Week Evaluation Questionnaire

Did you accomplish your goal of the week? Check "yes" or "no" below and jot down answers to the related questions in full or in point form.

☐   YES   Congratulations: your goal was realistic.

What do you think made you successful at accomplishing your goal?

What have you learned about yourself and your abilities?

☐   NO   Consolation: your goal may have been too difficult to realize this week.

1. What barriers prevented you from accomplishing your goal?

2. What changes will you make to your goal so that you will be successful next time?

CASE STUDY Andrea's Program

Keeping Motivated

At the end of the week, Andrea looked at her list of goals and realized that she had already attained some. "Hey," Andrea noticed, "I can walk quickly around the block without getting winded." She checked off that goal and read through the rest of the list. "These goals are all attainable. I can do it," she said smiling.

Andrea continued her healthy eating and regular physical activity. She even found herself walking to her friends' houses and the mall instead of taking the bus or getting a ride. When eating out, she found herself ordering a soup, salad, and milk, instead of a burger, fries, and a pop.

Her weight eventually began to decrease. Slowly, she could see her goal could be reached.

continued on page 288

Setting Rewards

When we think of rewarding a child for good behavior, the first thing that comes to most people's mind are food treats — chocolate or candy or some other less healthy food choice. Our tendency to buy treats to use rewards has created a market for the little candy gifts you see at the checkout of almost any type of store these days. Some people must have a mixed up idea when they show how they care about people by encouraging them to eat less healthy foods. We all know that it is hard to resist treat foods when they are in front of us, especially if they are given as presents. Reversing these habits will be quite a difficult task, but many children are just as excited to receive a toy, game, or other non-food items as rewards or gifts.

Working Toward a Reward

Even though praise is the best reward, sometimes having a prearranged reward can help children to push themselves to make an extra effort. Rewards are a great motivator, especially when your child chooses their reward. You may decide to reward your child when they accomplish certain program goals, especially the ones that take several weeks and lots of dedication and effort. For example, accomplishing a 5-kilometer race is an amazing feat for an overweight child and may deserve recognition with a very special reward.

Realistic Rewards

The rewards you give should suit your child's accomplishments. While praise should always be given, rewards must be decided carefully and, sometimes, strategically. If you reward your child with new shoes or clothes every time they eat enough fruit, they will quickly run out of closet space and you'll run out of money. Small rewards should be given more frequently when your child is starting the program, to give them extra encouragement to get through the first 5 weeks. As your child settles into the program, rewards should then be used when specific goals are met, especially challenging but achievable goals.

Pour on the Praise

The most important reward you can give is your praise for the positive health choices your child makes and the nutrition and activity goals they achieve. For most children, positive, encouraging words coming from people they look up to will make them feel much happier than the candy that might taste good for a few minutes while it is eaten.

Timing the Reward

To be most effective, rewards need to be timely and immediate. Give the reward shortly after the goal is tried or achieved. Never wait to give praise for a job well done. If you have promised your child a new bicycle for completing their first 5-kilometer race, go out that very day and buy it for them.

Not Helpful	Better	Big
Candy	Books	Bicycle
Chocolates	Magazines	In-line Skates
Chips	Board Games	Athletic Shoes
Video/Computer Games	Art Supplies	Sports Ball
Movies	Puzzles	Skipping Rope, Frisbee
Television	Clothing	Exercise Videos
		Special trip to the zoo, science center, ball game, museum, or amusement parks

Appropriate Rewards

Appropriate rewards for successes are any gifts or events that are related to activity. The following is a list of examples of rewards that are not helpful, with better choices recommended and 'big' choices suggested for exceptional accomplishments.

3-Day Nutrition and Activity Diary (Week 2)

For the second week of the program, after the goal of the week has been evaluated, you should complete a 3-day nutrition and activity diary. This will serve to show any progress made in the first week and help in setting goals for the next week. You may not need to complete nutrition and activity logs if you have become familiar with counting nutrition servings and activity durations of the various food types and activities.

3-Day Nutrition Log and Scorecard (Week 2)

Instructions

1. Complete a log of nutrition servings as you did in Week 1 for 3 days and calculate the average daily number of servings for each food type.
2. Now put the average serving numbers on to the following scorecard under the column labeled "Week 2: Servings" — as you did in Week 1.
3. Find out what levels you have achieved for Week 2 from the serving numbers — from red flags to gold levels — into the column labeled "Week 2: Level."
4. Copy the "start" level information established in the Week 1 Nutrition Scorecard into the column labeled "Week 1: Start Level."
5. Now compare the level for Week 1 and Week 2 to see your child's progress and the final goal. As the program progresses week by week, you will set progressive goals, moving, for example, from copper to bronze in the first week.

Nutrition Scorecard: Week 2

Food Group	Week 2 Servings	Week 2 Level	Week 1 Start Level	Program Levels
Wholesome Foods				
Vegetables	☐ ☐ ☐ ☐ ☐ ☐ ☐	☐ Copper ☐ Bronze ☐ Silver ☐ Gold	☐ Copper ☐ Bronze ☐ Silver ☐ Gold	Copper: 1-2 Bronze: 3-4 Silver: 5 **Gold: 6+**
Fruit	☐ ☐ ☐	☐ Copper ☐ Bronze ☐ Silver ☐ Gold	☐ Copper ☐ Bronze ☐ Silver ☐ Gold	Copper: 0 Bronze: 1 Silver: 2 **Gold: 3**
Whole Grains	☐ ☐ ☐ ☐ ☐ ☐	☐ Copper ☐ Bronze ☐ Silver ☐ Gold	☐ Copper ☐ Bronze ☐ Silver ☐ Gold	Copper: 1-2 Bronze: 3 Silver: 4 **Gold: 5+**
Legumes, Nuts, Seeds	☐ ☐	☐ Copper ☐ Bronze ☐ Silver ☐ Gold	☐ Copper ☐ Bronze ☐ Silver ☐ Gold	Copper: 0 Bronze: 1 Silver: 2 **Gold: 3**
Fish, Poultry, Eggs, Lean Meat	☐ ☐ ☐	☐ Copper ☐ Bronze ☐ Silver ☐ Gold	☐ Copper ☐ Bronze ☐ Silver ☐ Gold	Copper: 0 Bronze: 1 Silver: 1-2 **Gold: 2-3**
Calcium Sources	⚑ ☐ ☐ ☐ ☐	☐ Red Flag ☐ Copper ☐ Bronze ☐ Silver ☐ Gold	☐ Red Flag ☐ Copper ☐ Bronze ☐ Silver ☐ Gold	Red Flag: 0 Copper: 1 Bronze: 2 Silver: 3 **Gold: 4**

Nutrition Scorecard: Week 2 (cont.)				
Food Group	**Week 2 Servings**	**Week 2 Level**	**Week 1 Start Level**	**Program Levels**
Processed Foods				
Refined Starch Products	☐ ☐ ☐ ☐ ☐ ⚑	☐ Gold ☐ Silver ☐ Bronze ☐ Copper ☐ Red Flag	☐ Gold ☐ Silver ☐ Bronze ☐ Copper ☐ Red Flag	**Gold: 0-1** Silver: 2 Bronze: 3 Copper: 4 Red Flag: 5+
Soft Drinks, Fruit Drinks	☐ ☐ ☐ ☐ ⚑	☐ Gold ☐ Silver ☐ Bronze ☐ Copper ☐ Red Flag	☐ Gold ☐ Silver ☐ Bronze ☐ Copper ☐ Red Flag	**Gold: 0-1** Silver: 2 Bronze: 3 Copper: 4 Red Flag: 5+
Other Sugar and Saturated Fat Foods	Total number of "other" foods: ☐ ☐ ☐ ☐ ☐ ⚑	☐ Gold ☐ Silver ☐ Bronze ☐ Copper ☐ Red Flag	☐ Gold ☐ Silver ☐ Bronze ☐ Copper ☐ Red Flag	**Gold: 0** Silver: 1-2 Bronze: 3-4 Copper: 5-6 Red Flag: 6+

3-Day Activity Log and Scorecard

Instructions

1. Complete a log of activities as you did in Week 1 for 3 days and calculate the average daily minutes for each type of activity.
2. Now write down the amount of time spent on a average day on to the scorecard under the column labeled "Week 2: Time Spent" — as you did in Week 1.
3. Find out what levels you have achieved for Week 2 from the average minutes per day – from red flags to gold levels – into the column labeled "Week 2: Level."
4. Copy the "start" level information established in the Week 1 Activity Scorecard into the column labeled "Week 1: Start Level."
5. Now compare the level for Week 1 and Week 2 to see your child's progress and the final goal. As the program progresses week-by-week, you will set progressive goals, moving, for example, from copper to bronze in the first week.

Activity Scorecard: Week 2

Type of Activity	Week 2 Time Spent (Duration in Minutes)	Week 2 Level	Week 1 Start Level	Program Level (minutes/day)
Moderate	Minutes:	☐ First Steps ☐ Copper ☐ Bronze ☐ Silver ☐ Gold	☐ First Steps ☐ Copper ☐ Bronze ☐ Silver ☐ Gold	First: 0-20 Copper: 21-30 Bronze: 31-40 Silver: 41-59 **Gold: 60+**
Vigorous	Minutes:	☐ First Steps ☐ Copper ☐ Bronze ☐ Silver ☐ Gold	☐ First Steps ☐ Copper ☐ Bronze ☐ Silver ☐ Gold	First: 0-10 Copper: 11-15 Bronze: 16-20 Silver: 21-29 **Gold: 30+**
Screen Time	Minutes:	☐ Gold ☐ Silver ☐ Bronze ☐ Copper ☐ Red Flag	☐ Gold ☐ Silver ☐ Bronze ☐ Copper ☐ Red Flag	**Gold: <60** Silver: 60-90 Bronze: 91-120 Copper: 121-150 Red Flag: >150

Stage 2 Review (Week 2)

☐ Goal of the Week Worksheet
☐ Goal of the Week Evaluation Questionnaire
☐ 3-Day Nutrition Diary: Log and Scorecard
☐ 3-Day Activity Diary: Log and Scorecard

STAGE 3

Building Up Goals and Rewards (Week 3-4)

Just because your child is successful at accomplishing their chosen program goal for the week does not mean that they drop that goal after the week is through. If your child chose "Eat more fruit this week" as their program goal and they were successful, they should try to keep eating the same amount of fruit regularly for every week after that, not just as part of a week-long exercise. By building up goal upon goal, week after week, a healthy weight will be achieved.

To see the effect of these weekly accomplishments of nutrition and activity goals, you can now turn back to the 3-Day Nutrition Diary and the 3-Day Activity Diary to see if your child has moved closer to the Gold level of healthy weight and good health. Every two weeks, you can return to the height, weight, and target weight chart to see if any changes can be seen.

Stage 3 Preview (Week 3-4)

☐ Goal of the Week Worksheet
☐ Goal of the Week Evaluation Questionnaire
☐ 3-Day Nutrition Diary: Log and Scorecard
☐ 3-Day Activity Diary: Log and Scorecard
☐ Height, Weight and Target Weight Chart

Setting New Goals

You can use the nutrition and activity scorecards to target future goal setting to the specific categories of nutrition and activity where improvements still need to be made. The aim will be to raise a food group or activity category from a bronze to a silver level, for example, then on to the gold level.

Suppose your child had a starting level of bronze in the fruit category. This means that during the assessment, they normally ate 1 serving of fruit a day. If they chose to improve their program level for fruit intake this week by eating an extra serving each day, they would reach the silver level. If they added another serving of fruit next week to the two they are now already having, they would reach the gold level. Their goal of the week would be to eat three servings of fruit per day. However, they might personalize that program goal, or they might focus on another food group for attention and begin their progress toward the gold level.

Keep It Simple
Continue to choose personalized program goals that are within reach. You want your child to be successful right away, not to reach the gold level necessarily the second or even third or fourth week. Remember that this is your child's own program and it should be used at their own pace. You are there to guide them and encourage them.

Goal of the Week
From your copies of Goal of the Week Worksheets, complete at least two worksheets, one a nutrition goal (knowledge or action), the other an activity goal (knowledge or action). You may find at this stage your child is ready to tackle more than two goals during a single week. However, be careful not to overload your child; or they may burn out or not be as successful, and then get discouraged. Setting goals should not create anxiety and worry or stress.

Goal of the Week Worksheet and Evaluation Questionnaire (Week 3-4)

Instructions
1. Look at the program level your child achieved in each category of nutrition and activity from the Week 1 and Week 2 nutrition and activity diary scorecards.
2. Choose at least one specific nutrition category and one specific activity category that needs to be improved.
3. Create personalized goal statements for each category chosen and complete a Goal of the Week Worksheet.
4. Complete a Goal of the Week Evaluation Questionnaire at the end of the week.
5. Aim to maintain, if not better, the same level your child achieved in all categories the previous week and to reach higher levels in new categories by achieving the new goals of the week they have set for next week. In this way, your child will always be improving their nutrition and activity level.

Nutrition Scorecard: Week 3 & 4

Food Group	Week 1 Start Level	Week 2 Servings Level	Week 3 Servings Level	Week 4 Servings Level	Gold Standard Servings per Day
Wholesome Foods					
Vegetables	☐ Copper ☐ Bronze ☐ Silver ☐ Gold	☐ Copper ☐ Bronze ☐ Silver ☐ Gold	☐ Copper ☐ Bronze ☐ Silver ☐ Gold	☐ Copper ☐ Bronze ☐ Silver ☐ Gold	Copper: 1-2 Bronze: 3-4 Silver: 5 **Gold: 6+**
Fruit	☐ Copper ☐ Bronze ☐ Silver ☐ Gold	☐ Copper ☐ Bronze ☐ Silver ☐ Gold	☐ Copper ☐ Bronze ☐ Silver ☐ Gold	☐ Copper ☐ Bronze ☐ Silver ☐ Gold	Copper: 0 Bronze: 1 Silver: 2 **Gold: 3**
Whole Grains	☐ Copper ☐ Bronze ☐ Silver ☐ Gold	☐ Copper ☐ Bronze ☐ Silver ☐ Gold	☐ Copper ☐ Bronze ☐ Silver ☐ Gold	☐ Copper ☐ Bronze ☐ Silver ☐ Gold	Copper: 1-2 Bronze: 3 Silver: 4 **Gold: 5+**
Legumes, Nuts, Seeds	☐ Copper ☐ Bronze ☐ Silver ☐ Gold	☐ Copper ☐ Bronze ☐ Silver ☐ Gold	☐ Copper ☐ Bronze ☐ Silver ☐ Gold	☐ Copper ☐ Bronze ☐ Silver ☐ Gold	Copper: 0 Bronze: 1 Silver: 2 **Gold: 3**
Fish, Poultry, Eggs, Lean Meat	☐ Copper ☐ Bronze ☐ Silver ☐ Gold	☐ Copper ☐ Bronze ☐ Silver ☐ Gold	☐ Copper ☐ Bronze ☐ Silver ☐ Gold	☐ Copper ☐ Bronze ☐ Silver ☐ Gold	Copper: 0 Bronze: 1 Silver: 1-2 **Gold: 2-3**
Calcium Sources	☐ Red Flag ☐ Copper ☐ Bronze ☐ Silver ☐ Gold	☐ Red Flag ☐ Copper ☐ Bronze ☐ Silver ☐ Gold	☐ Red Flag ☐ Copper ☐ Bronze ☐ Silver ☐ Gold	☐ Red Flag ☐ Copper ☐ Bronze ☐ Silver ☐ Gold	Red Flag: <2 Copper: <1 Bronze: 1 Silver: 2 **Gold: 3-4**
Processed Foods					
Refined Starch Products	☐ Gold ☐ Silver ☐ Bronze ☐ Copper ☐ Red Flag	☐ Gold ☐ Silver ☐ Bronze ☐ Copper ☐ Red Flag	☐ Gold ☐ Silver ☐ Bronze ☐ Copper ☐ Red Flag	☐ Gold ☐ Silver ☐ Bronze ☐ Copper ☐ Red Flag	**Gold: 0-1** Silver: 2 Bronze: 3 Copper: 4 Red Flag: 5+

Nutrition Scorecard: Week 3 & 4 (cont.)

Food Group	Week 1 Start Level	Week 2 Servings Level	Week 3 Servings Level	Week 4 Servings Level	Gold Standard Servings per Day
Processed Foods					
Soft Drinks, Fruit Drinks	□ Gold □ Silver □ Bronze □ Copper □ Red Flag	□ Gold □ Silver □ Bronze □ Copper □ Red Flag	□ Gold □ Silver □ Bronze □ Copper □ Red Flag	□ Gold □ Silver □ Bronze □ Copper □ Red Flag	**Gold: 0-1** Silver: 2 Bronze: 3 Copper: 4 Red Flag: 5+
Other Sugar and Saturated Fat Foods	□ Gold □ Silver □ Bronze □ Copper □ Red Flag	□ Gold □ Silver □ Bronze □ Copper □ Red Flag	□ Gold □ Silver □ Bronze □ Copper □ Red Flag	□ Gold □ Silver □ Bronze □ Copper □ Red Flag	**Gold: 0** Silver: 1-2 Bronze: 3-4 Copper: 5-6 Red Flag: 6+

Activity Scorecard: Week 3 & 4

Type of Activity	Week 1 Start Level	Week 2 Minutes Level	Week 3 Minutes Level	Week 4 Minutes Level	Gold Standard Minutes Per Day
Wholesome Foods					
Moderate	□ First Steps □ Copper □ Bronze □ Silver □ Gold	□ First Steps □ Copper □ Bronze □ Silver □ Gold	□ First Steps □ Copper □ Bronze □ Silver □ Gold	□ First Steps □ Copper □ Bronze □ Silver □ Gold	First: 0-20 Copper: 21-30 Bronze: 31-40 Silver: 41-50 **Gold: 60+**
Vigorous	□ First Steps □ Copper □ Bronze □ Silver □ Gold	□ First Steps □ Copper □ Bronze □ Silver □ Gold	□ First Steps □ Copper □ Bronze □ Silver □ Gold	□ First Steps □ Copper □ Bronze □ Silver □ Gold	First: 0-10 Copper: 11-15 Bronze: 16-20 Silver: 21-25 **Gold: 30+**
Screen Time	□ Gold □ Silver □ Bronze □ Copper □ Red Flag	□ Gold □ Silver □ Bronze □ Copper □ Red Flag	□ Gold □ Silver □ Bronze □ Copper □ Red Flag	□ Gold □ Silver □ Bronze □ Copper □ Red Flag	**Gold: <60** Silver: 61-90 Bronze: 91-120 Copper: 121-150 Red Flag: >150

Height, Weight and Target Weight Measurements

As another way of checking on progress toward a healthy weight, measure your child's current height, current weight and target weight, then record it on the following chart. Make the measurements in Week 4 and every second week after that.

Instructions
1. Transfer the height, weight, target weight and weight difference measurements from Week 1 to the Week 4 chart.
2. Use the same day of the week as you did in Week 1. Record the date.
3. Measure your child's height. Record the measurement in feet and inches or centimeters as chosen for recording height.
4. Measure your child's weight and record it. Record the measurement in pounds or kilograms. Always try to use the same weight scale.
5. Calculate your child's target weight using the body mass index (BMI) charts in Chapter 2, "How Do I Know If My Child Is Overweight?" (page 61)
6. Subtract your child's weight from the target weight and record the difference. This difference then becomes the total weight loss goal.

Height, Weight, and Target Weight Chart				
Date	**Height**	**Weight**	**Target Weight**	**Difference**
Week 1 Date:				
Week 4 Date:				

Stage 3 Review (Week 3-4)
☐ Goal of the Week Worksheet
☐ Goal of the Week Evaluation Questionnaire
☐ 3-Day Nutrition Diary: Log and Scorecard
☐ 3-Day Activity Diary: Log and Scorecard
☐ Height, Weight and Target Weight Chart

STAGE 4

Maintaining Progress (Beyond Week 4)

After the first 4 weeks of the program, the program requires less paperwork. Although you will continue to set and assess goals weekly and measure height and weight every other week, nutrition and activity logs and scorecards can be completed monthly. If you and your child feel that it is more helpful to keep track more often than every 4 weeks, that is perfectly fine. Some children and parents enjoy keeping records.

Weekly

Goal of the Week Worksheet and Evaluation Questionnaire

Continue the process of setting new knowledge or action nutrition and activity goals each week using the Goal of the Week Worksheets and Evaluation Questionnaires. Use the monthly nutrition and activity score card levels to help determine the nutrition and activity categories that need to be improved. Take on two or more goals each week until the next monthly log and scorecard are recorded.

Monthly

3-Day Nutrition and Activity Diary Log and Scorecards

We recommend keeping the 3-day diary every 4 weeks now, although your child may decide that keeping them more or less frequently is more suitable. Since several weeks may pass without your child recording their nutrition and activity, they may drop down a level or two in some categories and not really know it. To deal with this, you and your child will have to decide if more frequent record-keeping will be helpful. Use Week 4 from the previous scorecard as your Month 1 level here.

Nutrition Scorecard: Month 1, 2, 3, 4						
Food Group	Start Level Daily Servings	Month 1 Daily Servings	Month 2 Daily Servings	Month 3 Daily Servings	Month 4 Daily Servings	Gold Standard
Wholesome Foods						
Vegetables	☐ Copper ☐ Bronze ☐ Silver ☐ Gold	☐ Copper ☐ Bronze ☐ Silver ☐ Gold	☐ Copper ☐ Bronze ☐ Silver ☐ Gold	☐ Copper ☐ Bronze ☐ Silver ☐ Gold	☐ Copper ☐ Bronze ☐ Silver ☐ Gold	Copper: 1-2 Bronze: 3-4 Silver: 5 **Gold: 6+**
Fruit	☐ Copper ☐ Bronze ☐ Silver ☐ Gold	☐ Copper ☐ Bronze ☐ Silver ☐ Gold	☐ Copper ☐ Bronze ☐ Silver ☐ Gold	☐ Copper ☐ Bronze ☐ Silver ☐ Gold	☐ Copper ☐ Bronze ☐ Silver ☐ Gold	Copper: 0 Bronze: 1 Silver: 2 **Gold: 3**
Whole Grains	☐ Copper ☐ Bronze ☐ Silver ☐ Gold	☐ Copper ☐ Bronze ☐ Silver ☐ Gold	☐ Copper ☐ Bronze ☐ Silver ☐ Gold	☐ Copper ☐ Bronze ☐ Silver ☐ Gold	☐ Copper ☐ Bronze ☐ Silver ☐ Gold	Copper: 1-2 Bronze: 3 Silver: 4 **Gold: 5+**
Legumes, Nuts, Seeds	☐ Copper ☐ Bronze ☐ Silver ☐ Gold	☐ Copper ☐ Bronze ☐ Silver ☐ Gold	☐ Copper ☐ Bronze ☐ Silver ☐ Gold	☐ Copper ☐ Bronze ☐ Silver ☐ Gold	☐ Copper ☐ Bronze ☐ Silver ☐ Gold	Copper: 0 Bronze: 1 Silver: 2 **Gold: 3**
Fish, Poultry, Eggs, Lean Meat	☐ Copper ☐ Bronze ☐ Silver ☐ Gold	☐ Copper ☐ Bronze ☐ Silver ☐ Gold	☐ Copper ☐ Bronze ☐ Silver ☐ Gold	☐ Copper ☐ Bronze ☐ Silver ☐ Gold	☐ Copper ☐ Bronze ☐ Silver ☐ Gold	Copper: 0 Bronze: 1 Silver: 1-2 **Gold: 2-3**
Calcium Sources	☐ Red Flag ☐ Copper ☐ Bronze ☐ Silver ☐ Gold	☐ Red Flag ☐ Copper ☐ Bronze ☐ Silver ☐ Gold	☐ Red Flag ☐ Copper ☐ Bronze ☐ Silver ☐ Gold	☐ Red Flag ☐ Copper ☐ Bronze ☐ Silver ☐ Gold	☐ Red Flag ☐ Copper ☐ Bronze ☐ Silver ☐ Gold	Red Flag: <2 Copper: <1 Bronze: 1 Silver: 2 **Gold: 3-4**

Nutrition Scorecard: Month 1, 2, 3, 4 (cont.)

Food Group	Start Level Daily Servings	Month 1 Daily Servings	Month 2 Daily Servings	Month 3 Daily Servings	Month 4 Daily Servings	Gold Standard
Processed Foods						
Refined Starch Products	□ Gold □ Silver □ Bronze □ Copper □ Red Flag	□ Gold □ Silver □ Bronze □ Copper □ Red Flag	□ Gold □ Silver □ Bronze □ Copper □ Red Flag	□ Gold □ Silver □ Bronze □ Copper □ Red Flag	□ Gold □ Silver □ Bronze □ Copper □ Red Flag	**Gold: 0-1** Silver: 2 Bronze: 3 Copper: 4 Red Flag: 5+
Soft Drinks, Fruit Drinks	□ Gold □ Silver □ Bronze □ Copper □ Red Flag	□ Gold □ Silver □ Bronze □ Copper □ Red Flag	□ Gold □ Silver □ Bronze □ Copper □ Red Flag	□ Gold □ Silver □ Bronze □ Copper □ Red Flag	□ Gold □ Silver □ Bronze □ Copper □ Red Flag	**Gold: 0-2** Silver: 2 Bronze: 3 Copper: 4 Red Flag: 5+
Other Sugar and Saturated Fat Foods	□ Gold □ Silver □ Bronze □ Copper □ Red Flag	□ Gold □ Silver □ Bronze □ Copper □ Red Flag	□ Gold □ Silver □ Bronze □ Copper □ Red Flag	□ Gold □ Silver □ Bronze □ Copper □ Red Flag	□ Gold □ Silver □ Bronze □ Copper □ Red Flag	**Gold: 0** Silver: 1-2 Bronze: 3-4 Copper: 5-6 Red Flag: 6+

Activity Scorecard: Month 1, 2, 3, 4

Type of Activity	Start Level Week 1	Week 2 Daily Minutes	Month 2 Daily Minutes	Month 3 Daily Minutes	Month 4 Daily Minutes	Gold Standard (minutes/day)
Moderate	□ First Steps □ Copper □ Bronze □ Silver □ Gold	□ First Steps □ Copper □ Bronze □ Silver □ Gold	□ First Steps □ Copper □ Bronze □ Silver □ Gold	□ First Steps □ Copper □ Bronze □ Silver □ Gold	□ First Steps □ Copper □ Bronze □ Silver □ Gold	First: 0–20 Copper: 21-30 Bronze: 31-40 Silver: 41-50 **Gold: 60+**
Vigorous	□ First Steps □ Copper □ Bronze □ Silver □ Gold	□ First Steps □ Copper □ Bronze □ Silver □ Gold	□ First Steps □ Copper □ Bronze □ Silver □ Gold	□ First Steps □ Copper □ Bronze □ Silver □ Gold	□ First Steps □ Copper □ Bronze □ Silver □ Gold	First: 0–10 Copper: 11-15 Bronze: 16-20 Silver: 21-25 **Gold: 30+**
Screen Time	□ Gold □ Silver □ Bronze □ Copper □ Red Flag	□ Gold □ Silver □ Bronze □ Copper □ Red Flag	□ Gold □ Silver □ Bronze □ Copper □ Red Flag	□ Gold □ Silver □ Bronze □ Copper □ Red Flag	□ Gold □ Silver □ Bronze □ Copper □ Red Flag	**Gold: <60** Silver: 61-90 Bronze: 91-20 Copper: 121-150 Red Flag: >150

Q: How do we deal with setbacks?

A: Giving your children control of the program by allowing them to choose their own goals is an approach that will increase the likelihood that they will accomplish those goals. Even so, there will be times when they are unable to accomplish a goal that they have set. When this happens, it is important that your child does not feel guilty. To prevent feelings of guilt, help them to understand the reason they were not successful. Sometimes there will be a specific uncontrollable barrier that got in the way of their success.

Review with your child the factors that they may have control over and the ones they do not. For the factors that they have control over, help your child figure out how they can deal with them differently the next time. For factors they cannot control, help your child figure out alternatives for getting around them.

Don't blame your child and always make sure that they do not feel guilty about any setbacks. Give praise for any improvements they make, but don't criticize or blame your child for setbacks.

CASE STUDY Andrea's Program

Slow Progress

After a month, Andrea was starting to get frustrated with her lifestyle change and wondered if it was even worth it. One morning before school, Andrea weighed herself and found that her weight had not changed despite her regular physical activity and healthy eating. That day at school, out of frustration, she decided to eat whatever she wanted for lunch. She opted for French fries, onion rings, chips, and a large pop.

After school, she went to her mother and explained her dilemma. She admitted that due to her frustrations with her lack of progress, she had eaten a less healthy lunch. Her mother had seen all of Andrea's hard work and reassured her that one slip was not the end of the world, and that everyone had setbacks. Her mother explained that the exercise may have been causing her to gain lean muscle while she is losing fat, and that muscle weighs more that fat.

Then her mother went and got Andrea's favorite pair of sweat pants and told her to try them on. Andrea put them on. "Wow," she said when she realized that the waistband of the pants, which used to be tight, were now looser. After that, whenever she felt that she was making no progress, she put on her old sweat pants and read over the goals she had accomplished.

continued on page 288

Biweekly (Every 2 Weeks)

Height, Weight and Target Weight Measurements

Continue to make these measurements every 2 weeks for the next 6 months to 1 year. The difference between your child's actual weight and target weight should decrease progressively though gradually if The Healthy Weight Program is working effectively.

After several months of the program, we recommend that you review not only your child's, but also your family's progress. You might want to complete the Family Nutrition and Activity Habits Worksheet and the Child's Nutrition and Activity Habits Worksheet again to see how far everyone has come since the assessment in Week 1. Continue to be patient. Be caring. Be positive. Getting a healthy weight for your child and family is worth the effort.

Height, Weight, and Target Weight Chart				
Date	Height	Weight	Target Weight	Difference
Week 1 Date:				
Week 4 Date:				
Week 6 Date:				
Week 8 Date:				
Week 10 Date:				
Week 12 Date:				

CASE STUDY Andrea's Program

A Good Day in Dance Class

"Andrea, I hear that Anna is teaching a fun hip-hop class at the community center today. We should definitely check it out!" Andrea had heard about the special class. "Sounds like a great plan, Robyn!" Andrea exclaimed, but inside she felt nervous. She had definitely become more fit since her first experience in the dance class and she did feel better about herself.

Andrea decided that she would go, but would take a spot at the back of the room. At least then if she felt short of breath or struggled with the class, no one would be able to see her. As the class progressed, Andrea realized how comfortable she was. She was impressed by how much control she had over her body, even though Anna was teaching a new dance routine. She was feeling confident in her dancing abilities and it showed. After 15 minutes into the class, Andrea still hadn't even begun to sweat or lose her breath. Andrea was feeling great and decided to move to the front of the dance class with all of her friends.

"Great job, Andrea!" Anna, the dance teacher, yelled. "Hold the stretch for 5 more seconds!" Anna instructed. However, this time Andrea was able to hold it for 10 seconds. Andrea was extremely proud of her improved fitness achievements, and as the dance class ended, she found herself eagerly awaiting the next one!

Andrea sat on her bed after school and stared at herself in last year's class photo, reminiscing about the one dance class that changed everything for her. It had all seemed so long ago. Her gaze shifted to her full-length bedside mirror, noticing how much leaner and fitter her body looked. She wasn't skinny by any means, but that was never her goal. Her physique and mood had improved so much since last year.

After examining herself with satisfaction, she crossed the room and entered the bathroom, smiling and humming tunefully. She pulled the weigh scale out of the cupboard; it had been months since she had used it. Her grin broadened as she saw that her weight was within the healthy range for her age and height. Just then, she heard the front door of the house close. Her mom was home from work. Andrea sprinted down the stairs and threw her arms around her mom. "Thank you so much!" she whispered in her mother's ear.

Healthy Weight Resources

The United States of America

USDA Food and Nutrition Service
*A division of the USDA committed to
providing children and low-income families
with access to food and nutrition education.*
3101 Park Center Drive, Room 926
Alexandria, VA 22302
Tel: 703-305-2062
www.fns.usda.gov/fns/

Center for Nutrition Policy and Promotion
*A division of the USDA dedicated to
developing and disseminating sound dietary
advice linking scientific research to the
nutrition needs of consumers.*
3101 Park Center Drive, Room 1034
Alexandria, VA 22302-1594
Tel: 703-305-7600

**Steps to a Healthier You —
USDA Food Pyramid**
*All about the new USDA Food Pyramid and
how to incorporate it into your daily
routine.*
USDA Food and Nutrition Service
3101 Park Center Drive, Room 926
Alexandria, VA 22302
Tel: 703-305-2062
www.mypyramid.gov/

American Dietetic Association
*National association committed to
addressing issues in obesity, aging, dietary
supplements, food supply and genetics
within a context of helping people lead
healthy lives.*
120 South Riverside Plaza, Suite 2000
Chicago, IL 60606-6995
Toll Free: 800-877-1600
http://www.eatright.org/Public/

Food and Nutrition Information Center
*Division of the United States Department of
Agriculture dedicated to the dissemination
of food and nutrition information.*
Agricultural Research Service, USDA
National Agricultural Library, Room 105
10301 Baltimore Avenue
Beltsville, MD 20705-2351
Tel: 301-504-5719
E-mail: fnic@nal.usda.gov
www.nal.usda.gov/fnic/

**Harvard School of Public Health —
The Nutrition Source**
*A collaborative effort between the
department of nutrition and the school of
public health to provide concise nutritional
information to both health professionals
and the general public.*
677 Huntington Avenue
Boston, MA 02115
www.hsph.harvard.edu/
nutritionsource/index.html
Tel: (617) 432-4388

American Obesity Association
*Main focus on education and prevention of
obesity, especially among children.*
1250 24th Street NW, Suite 300
Washington, DC 20037
Tel: 202-776-7711
E-mail: webmaster@obesity.org
www.obesity.org/

**Center for Disease Control —
Nutrition and Physical Activity Program**
*Resources and information about physical
activity and good nutrition that are key
factors in leading a healthy lifestyle and
reducing chronic illnesses.*
4770 Buford Highway, NE, MS/K-24
Atlanta, GA 30341-3717
Tel: 770-488-5820
E-mail: ccdinfo@cdc.gov.
www.cdc.gov/nccdphp/dnpa/
index.htm

Canada

Health Canada — Food and Nutrition
Improving and protecting the health of Canadians through promotion of good nutrition.
Health Canada Headquarters
A.L. 0900C2
Ottawa, Canada
K1A 0K9
Toll Free: 1-866-225-0709
www.hc-sc.gc.ca/english/lifestyles/
food_nutr.html

Dietitians of Canada
Representative for dietitians across Canada and promotes health and well-being through healthy eating.
480 University Avenue, Suite 604
Toronto, ON M5G 1V2
Tel: 416-596-0857
www.dietitians.ca

The Canadian Council of Food and Nutrition
To communicate nutritional information and make the eating experience a positive one.
3800 Steeles Avenue West, Suite 301A
Woodbridge, ON L4L 4G9
Tel: 905-265-9124
www.ccfn.ca/

Office of Nutrition Policy and Promotion
Promoting nutritional health and wellbeing for Canadians.
Health Canada
Tower A, Qualicum Towers
2936 Baseline Road, 3rd Floor, A.L. 3303D
Ottawa, ON K1A 0K9
Tel: 613-957-8329
www.hc-sc.gc.ca/hpfb-dgpsa/
onpp-bppn/index_e.html

Canadian Food Inspection Agency
Enforcement of food safety and nutritional quality standards set by Health Canada.
59 Camelot Drive
Ottawa, ON K1A 0Y9
Tel: 613-225-2342
www.inspection.gc.ca

Canadian Institute of Child Health
Solely dedicated to improving children's health and educating professionals.
384 Bank Street, Suite 300
Ottawa, ON K2P 1Y4
Tel: 613-230-8838
www.cich.ca

Canadian Paediatric Society
Educating parents and health professionals alike on children's health.
2305 St. Laurent Boulevard
Ottawa, ON K1G 4J8
Tel: 613-526-9397
www.cps.ca

Health Canada — Physical Activity Unit
A part of the Public Health Agency of Canada, this site is concerned with promotion of physical activity among children and youth.
Jeanne Mance Building, 7th Floor
A.L. 1907C1
Tunney's Pasture
Ottawa, ON K1A 0K9
Tel: 613-941-3109
www.hc-sc.gc.ca/hppb/paguide/child_youth/
index.html

Safe Kids Canada
A branch of the Hospital for Sick Children dedicated to preventing unintentional injury in children.
180 Dundas Street West
Toronto, ON
Toll Free: 888-SAFE TIPS (723-3847)
www.safekidscanada.ca

References

Electronic Citations

American College of Sports Medicine
www.acsm.org/

American Obesity Association — Obesity
Prevention
www.obesity.org/subs/childhood/prevention.shtml

American Children's Diets Not Making the Grade
www.ers.usda.gov/publications/foodreview/
may2001/frv24I2b.pdf

America's Eating Habits: Changes and
Consequences. U.S. Department of Agriculture,
Economic Research Service, Food and Rural
Economics Division. Agriculture Information
Bulletin No. 750
www.ers.usda.gov/publications/aib750/aib750.pdf

Health Canada — Healthy Living
www.hc-sc.gc.ca/english/lifestyles/index.html

Health Indicators 2002
Statistics Canada, The Daily — Wednesday,
May 8, 2002
www.statcan.ca/Daily/English/020508/
td020508.htm

Parent and child factors associated with youth
obesity
Statistics Canada, The Daily — Monday,
November 3, 2003
www.statcan.ca/Daily/English/031103/
d031103a.htm

United States Department of Agriculture
www.usda.gov/wps/portal/usdahome

USDA National Nutrient Database for Standard
Reference
www.nal.usda.gov/fnic/foodcomp/search/

Journals/Reports

Adams GR, Hicken MS, Slalehi M. Socialization
of the physical attractiveness stereotype: Parental
expectations and verbal behaviors. Int J Psychol
1988;23:137-149.

Adelman RD, Restaino IG, Alon US, Blowey DL.
Proteinuria and focal segmental glomerulosclerosis
in severely obese adolescents. J Pediatr 2001;
138(4):481-485.

Andersen RE, Crespo CJ, Bartlett SJ, Cheskin LJ,
Pratt M. Relationship of physical activity and
television watching with body weight and level of
fatness among children: Results from the Third
National Health and Nutrition Examination
Survey. JAMA 1998;279(12):938-942.

Balcer LJ, Liu GT, Forman S, Pun K, Volpe NJ,
Galetta SL et al. Idiopathic intracranial
hypertension: Relation of age and obesity in
children. Neurology 1999;52(4):870-872.

Ball GD, McCargar LJ. Childhood obesity in
Canada: a review of prevalence estimates and risk
factors for cardiovascular diseases and type 2
diabetes. Can J Appl Physiol 2003;28(1):117-140.

Bao W, Srinivasan SR, Wattigney WA, Berenson
GS. Persistence of multiple cardiovascular risk
clustering related to syndrome X from childhood
to young adulthood. The Bogalusa Heart Study.
Arch Intern Med 1994;154(16):1842-1847.

Barsh GS, Farooqi IS, O'Rahilly S. Genetics of
body-weight regulation. Nature 2000;404(6778):
644-651.

Belamarich PF, Luder E, Kattan M, Mitchell H,
Islam S, Lynn H et al. Do obese inner-city
children with asthma have more symptoms than
non-obese children with asthma? Pediatrics
2000;106(6):1436-1441.

Bergmann KE, Bergmann RL, von Kries R, Bohm
O, Richter R, Dudenhausen JW et al. Early
determinants of childhood overweight and
adiposity in a birth cohort study: Role of breastfeeding. Int J Obes Relat Metab Disord
2003;27(2):162-172.

Berkey CS, Rockett HR, Field AE, Gillman MW,
Frazier AL, Camargo CA, Jr. et al. Activity,
dietary intake, and weight changes in a
longitudinal study of preadolescent and
adolescent boys and girls. Pediatrics
2000;105(4):E56.

Birch LL, Fisher JO. Mothers' child-feeding
practices influence daughters' eating and weight.
Am J Clin Nutr 2000;71(5):1054-1061.

Birch LL, Johnson SL, Andresen G, Peters JC,
Schulte MC. The variability of young children's
energy intake. N Engl J Med 1991;324(4):232-235.

Birch LL, McPhee L, Shoba BC, Pirok E, Steinberg L. What kind of exposure reduces children's food neophobia? Looking vs. tasting. Appetite 1987;9(3):171-178.

Borzekowski DL, Robinson TN. The 30-second effect: An experiment revealing the impact of television commercials on food preferences of preschoolers. J Am Diet Assoc 2001;101(1):42-46.

Bouchard C, Tremblay A. Genetic influences on the response of body fat and fat distribution to positive and negative energy balances in human identical twins. J Nutr 1997;127(5 Suppl):943S-947S.

Bouchard C, Tremblay A, Despres JP, Nadeau A, Lupien PJ, Theriault G et al. The response to long-term overfeeding in identical twins. N Engl J Med 1990;322(21):1477-1482.

Braet C, Mervielde I, Vandereycken W. Psychological aspects of childhood obesity: A controlled study in a clinical and nonclinical sample. J Pediatr Psychol 1997;22(1):59-71.

Brambilla P, Manzoni P, Sironi S, Simone P, Del Maschio A, di Natale B et al. Peripheral and abdominal adiposity in childhood obesity. Int J Obes Relat Metab Disord 1994;18(12):795-800.

Brylinskey JA, Moore JC. The identification of body build stereotypes in young children. J Res Pers 1994;(28):170-181.

Burke V, Beilin LJ, Dunbar D. Family lifestyle and parental body mass index as predictors of body mass index in Australian children: A longitudinal study. Int J Obes Relat Metab Disord 2001;25(2):147-157.

Caprio S, Hyman LD, McCarthy S, Lange R, Bronson M, Tamborlane WV. Fat distribution and cardiovascular risk factors in obese adolescent girls: Importance of the intraabdominal fat depot. Am J Clin Nutr 1996;64(1):12-17.

Caprio S, Tamborlane WV, Silver D, Robinson C, Leibel R, McCarthy S et al. Hyperleptinemia: An early sign of juvenile obesity. Relations to body fat depots and insulin concentrations. Am J Physiol 1996;271(3 Pt 1):E626-E630.

Cavadini C, Siega-Riz AM, Popkin BM. US adolescent food intake trends from 1965 to 1996. West J Med 2000;173(6):378-383.

Chinn S, Rona RJ. Prevalence and trends in overweight and obesity in three cross sectional studies of British Children, 1974-94. BMJ 2001;322(7277):24-26.

Cook S, Weitzman M, Auinger P, Nguyen M, Dietz WH. Prevalence of a metabolic syndrome phenotype in adolescents: findings from the third National Health and Nutrition Examination Survey, 1988-1994. Arch Pediatr Adolesc Med 2003;157(8):821-827.

Coon KA, Goldberg J, Rogers BL, Tucker KL. Relationships between use of television during meals and children's food consumption patterns. Pediatrics 2001;107(1):E7.

Cope MB, Fernandez JR, Allison DB. Genetic and Biological Risk Factors. In: Thompson JK, editor. Handbook of Eating Disorders and Obesity. Hoboken, NJ: John Wiley & Sons, Inc., 2004: 323-338.

Cramer P, Steinwert T. Thin is good, fat is bad: How early does it begin? Journal of Applied Developmental Psychology 1998;19(3):429-451.

Crandall CS. Prejudice against fat people: ideology and self-interest. J Pers Soc Psychol 1994;66(5): 882-894.

Crichlow RW, Seltzer MH, Jannetta PJ. Cholecystitis in adolescents. Am J Dig Dis 1972;17(1):68-72.

Davison KK, Birch LL. Weight status, parent reaction, and self-concept in five-year-old girls. Pediatrics 2001;107(1):46-53.

de Onis M, Blossner M. Prevalence and trends of overweight among preschool children in developing countries. Am J Clin Nutr 2000;72(4):1032-1039.

Dietz WH. Health consequences of obesity in youth: childhood predictors of adult disease. Pediatrics 1998;101(3 Pt 2):518-525.

Dowling AM, Steele JR, Baur LA. Does obesity influence foot structure and plantar pressure patterns in prepubescent children? Int J Obes Relat Metab Disord 2001;25(6):845-852.

DuRant RH, Baranowski T, Rhodes T, Gutin B, Thompson WO, Carroll R et al. Association among serum lipid and lipoprotein concentrations and physical activity, physical fitness, and body composition in young children. J Pediatr 1993;123(2):185-192.

Dyson LK. American cuisine in the 20th century. Food Review 2000; 23:2-7.

Ebbeling CB, Leidig MM, Sinclair KB, Hangen JP, Ludwig DS. A reduced-glycemic load diet in the treatment of adolescent obesity. Arch Pediatr Adolesc Med 2003;157(8):773-779.

Ebbeling CB, Pawlak DB, Ludwig DS. Childhood obesity: public-health crisis, common sense cure. Lancet 2002;360(9331):473-482.

Eisenberg ME, Neumark-Sztainer D, Story M. Associations of weight-based teasing and emotional well-being among adolescents. Arch Pediatr Adolesc Med 2003;157(8):733-738.

Epstein LH, Paluch RA, Gordy CC, Dorn J. Decreasing sedentary behaviors in treating pediatric obesity. Arch Pediatr Adolesc Med 2000;154(3):220-226.

Erickson SJ, Robinson TN, Haydel KF, Killen JD. Are overweight children unhappy?: Body mass index, depressive symptoms, and overweight concerns in elementary school children. Arch Pediatr Adolesc Med 2000;154(9):931-935.

Eriksson J, Forsen T, Osmond C, Barker D. Obesity from cradle to grave. Int J Obes Relat Metab Disord 2003;27(6):722-727.

Ferguson MA, Gutin B, Owens S, Litaker M, Tracy RP, Allison J. Fat distribution and hemostatic measures in obese children. Am J Clin Nutr 1998;67(6):1136-1140.

Figueroa-Munoz JI, Chinn S, Rona RJ. Association between obesity and asthma in 4-11 year old children in the UK. Thorax 2001;56(2):133-137.

Filozof C, Gonzalez C, Sereday M, Mazza C, Braguinsky J. Obesity prevalence and trends in Latin-American countries. Obes Rev 2001;2(2): 99-106.

Fisher J, Mitchell D, Smiciklas-Wright H, Birch L. Maternal milk consumption predicts the tradeoff between milk and soft drinks in young girls' diets. J Nutr 2001;131(2):246-250.

Fisher JO, Birch LL. Restricting access to foods and children's eating. Appetite 1999;32(3):405-419.

Fisher JO, Birch LL. Parents' restrictive feeding practices are associated with young girls' negative self-evaluation of eating. J Am Diet Assoc 2000;100(11):1341-1346.

Fisher JO, Mitchell DC, Smiciklas-Wright H, Birch LL. Parental influences on young girls' fruit and vegetable, micronutrient, and fat intakes. J Am Diet Assoc 2002;102(1):58-64.

Fogelholm M, Nuutinen O, Pasanen M, Myohanen E, Saatela T. Parent-child relationship of physical activity patterns and obesity. Int J Obes Relat Metab Disord 1999;23(12):1262-1268.

Ford ES, Galuska DA, Gillespie C, Will JC, Giles WH, Dietz WH. C-reactive protein and body mass index in children: findings from the Third National Health and Nutrition Examination Survey, 1988-1994. J Pediatr 2001;138(4):486-492.

Freedman DS, Dietz WH, Srinivasan SR, Berenson GS. The relation of overweight to cardiovascular risk factors among children and adolescents: the Bogalusa Heart Study. Pediatrics 1999;103(6 Pt 1):1175-1182.

French SA, Jeffery RW, Story M, Hannan P, Snyder MP. A pricing strategy to promote low-fat snack choices through vending machines. Am J Public Health 1997;87(5):849-851.

French SA, Story M, Jeffery RW. Environmental influences on eating and physical activity. Annu Rev Public Health 2001;22:309-335.

Gardner RM, Sorter RG, Friedman BN. Developmental changes in children's body images. J Soc Behav Pers 1997;12:1019-1036.

Gortmaker SL, Must A, Perrin JM, Sobol AM, Dietz WH. Social and economic consequences of overweight in adolescence and young adulthood. N Engl J Med 1993;329(14):1008-1012.

Gortmaker SL, Must A, Sobol AM, Peterson K, Colditz GA, Dietz WH. Television viewing as a cause of increasing obesity among children in the United States, 1986-1990. Arch Pediatr Adolesc Med 1996;150(4):356-362.

Goulding A, Jones IE, Taylor RW, Williams SM, Manning PJ. Bone mineral density and body composition in boys with distal forearm fractures: A dual-energy x-ray absorptiometry study. J Pediatr 2001;139(4):509-515.

Goulding A, Taylor RW, Jones IE, McAuley KA, Manning PJ, Williams SM. Overweight and obese children have low bone mass and area for their weight. Int J Obes Relat Metab Disord 2000;24(5):627-632.

Gutin B, Islam S, Treiber F, Smith C, Manos T. Fasting insulin concentration is related to cardiovascular reactivity to exercise in children. Pediatrics 1995;96(6):1123-1125.

Hainer V, Stunkard AJ, Kunesova M, Parizkova J, Stich V, Allison DB. Intrapair resemblance in very low calorie diet-induced weight loss in female obese identical twins. Int J Obes Relat Metab Disord 2000;24(8):1051-1057.

Harnack L, Stang J, Story M. Soft drink consumption among US children and adolescents: nutritional consequences. J Am Diet Assoc 1999;99(4):436-441.

Hayden-Wade HA. A proposed psychosocial consequences model of childhood obesity. Dissertation Abstracts International: Section B: The Sciences & Engineering 2002;63(3-B):1563.

Hill AJ, Silver EK. Fat, friendless and unhealthy: 9-year old children's perception of body shape stereotypes. Int J Obes Relat Metab Disord 1995;19(6):423-430.

Hill JO, Peters JC. Environmental contributions to the obesity epidemic. Science 1998;280(5368): 1371-1374.

Horgan KB, Choate M, Brownell K. Television food advertising: Targeting children in a toxic environment. In: D.G. Singer & J.L. Singer, ed. Handbook of Children and the Media. Thousand Oaks, CA: Sage, 2001:447-462.

Humphries MC, Gutin B, Barbeau P, Vemulapalli S, Allison J, Owens S. Relations of adiposity and effects of training on the left ventricle in obese youths. Med Sci Sports Exerc 2002;34(9):1428-1435.

Jeffery RW, French SA, Raether C, Baxter JE. An environmental intervention to increase fruit and salad purchases in a cafeteria. Prev Med 1994;23(6):788-792.

Johnson JG, Cohen P, Kasen S, Brook JS. Childhood adversities associated with risk for eating disorders or weight problems during adolescence or early adulthood. Am J Psychiatry 2002;159(3):394-400.

Kaplowitz PB, Slora EJ, Wasserman RC, Pedlow SE, Herman-Giddens ME. Earlier onset of puberty in girls: Relation to increased body mass index and race. Pediatrics 2001;108(2):347-353.

Katzmarzyk PT. The Canadian obesity epidemic, 1985-1998. CMAJ 2002;166(8):1039-1040.

Katzmarzyk PT, Gledhill N, Shephard RJ. The economic burden of physical inactivity in Canada. CMAJ 2000;163(11):1435-1440.

Katzmarzyk PT, Perusse L, Malina RM, Bergeron J, Despres JP, Bouchard C. Stability of indicators of the metabolic syndrome from childhood and adolescence to young adulthood: The Quebec Family Study. J Clin Epidemiol 2001;54(2): 190-195.

Kelsey JL, Acheson RM, Keggi KJ. The body build of patients with slipped capital femoral epiphysis. Am J Dis Child 1972;124(2):276-281.

Kelsey JL, Keggi KJ, Southwick WO. The incidence and distrubition of slipped capital femoral epiphysis in Connecticut and Southwestern United States. J Bone Joint Surg Am 1970;52(6):1203-1216.

Kimm SY, Glynn NW, Kriska AM, Barton BA, Kronsberg SS, Daniels SR et al. Decline in physical activity in black girls and white girls during adolescence. N Engl J Med 2002;347(10):709-715.

Kinugasa A, Tsunamoto K, Furukawa N, Sawada T, Kusunoki T, Shimada N. Fatty liver and its fibrous changes found in simple obesity of children. J Pediatr Gastroenterol Nutr 1984;3(3):408-414.

Klesges RC, Stein RJ, Eck LH, Isbell TR, Klesges LM. Parental influence on food selection in young children and its relationships to childhood obesity. Am J Clin Nutr 1991;53(4):859-864.

Kotz K, Story M. Food advertisements during children's Saturday morning television programming: Are they consistent with dietary recommendations? J Am Diet Assoc 1994;94:1296-1300.

Kraak V, Pelletier DL. The influence of commercialism on the food purchasing behavior of children and teenage youth. Fam Econ Nutr Rev 1998;11:15-24.

Kunkel D. Children and television advertising. Thousand Oaks, CA: Sage, 2001.

Latner JD, Stunkard AJ. Getting worse: The stigmatization of obese children. Obes Res 2003;11(3):452-456.

Levine J. Food industry marketing in elementary schools: Implications for school health professionals. J Sch Health 1999;69(7):290-291.

Lewis MK, Hill AJ. Food advertising on British children's television: A content analysis and experimental study with nine-year olds. Int J Obes Relat Metab Disord 1998;22(3):206-214.

Lissau I, Sorensen TI. Parental neglect during childhood and increased risk of obesity in young adulthood. Lancet 1994;343(8893):324-327.

Liu S, Willett WC, Stampfer MJ, Hu FB, Franz M, Sampson L et al. A prospective study of dietary glycemic load, carbohydrate intake, and risk of coronary heart disease in US women. Am J Clin Nutr 2000;71(6):1455-1461.

Loder RT, Aronson DD, Greenfield ML. The epidemiology of bilateral slipped capital femoral epiphysis. A study of children in Michigan. J Bone Joint Surg Am 1993;75(8):1141-1147.

Ludwig DS, Majzoub JA, Al Zahrani A, Dallal GE, Blanco I, Roberts SB. High glycemic index foods, overeating, and obesity. Pediatrics 1999;103(3):E26.

Ludwig DS, Peterson KE, Gortmaker SL. Relation between consumption of sugar-sweetened drinks and childhood obesity: A prospective, observational analysis. Lancet 2001; 57(9255):505-508.

Lytle LA, Himes JH, Feldman H, Zive M, Dwyer J, Hoelscher D et al. Nutrient intake over time in a multi-ethnic sample of youth. Public Health Nutr 2002;5(2):319-328.

Maes HH, Neale MC, Eaves LJ. Genetic and environmental factors in relative body weight and human adiposity. Behav Genet 1997;27(4): 325-351.

Magarey AM, Daniels LA, Boulton TJ. Prevalence of overweight and obesity in Australian children and adolescents: Reassessment of 1985 and 1995 data against new standard international definitions. Med J Aust 2001;174(11):561-564.

Mahoney LT, Burns TL, Stanford W, Thompson BH, Witt JD, Rost CA et al. Coronary risk factors measured in childhood and young adult life are associated with coronary artery calcification in young adults: The Muscatine Study. J Am Coll Cardiol 1996;27(2):277-284.

Mallory GB, Jr., Fiser DH, Jackson R. Sleep-associated breathing disorders in morbidly obese children and adolescents. J Pediatr 1989;115(6):892-897.

McCarthy HD, Ellis SM, Cole TJ. Central overweight and obesity in British youth aged 11-16 years: Cross sectional surveys of waist circumference. BMJ 2003;326(7390):624.

Mellbin T, Vuille JC. Further evidence of an association between psychosocial problems and increase in relative weight between 7 and 10 years of age. Acta Paediatr Scand 1989;78(4):576-580.

Mitchell BM, Gutin B, Kapuku G, Barbeau P, Humphries MC, Owens S et al. Left ventricular structure and function in obese adolescents: Relations to cardiovascular fitness, percent body fat, and visceral adiposity, and effects of physical training. Pediatrics 2002;109(5):E73.

Mo-suwan L, Lebel L, Puetpaiboon A, Junjana C. School performance and weight status of children and young adolescents in a transitional society in Thailand. Int J Obes Relat Metab Disord 1999;23(3):272-277.

Munoz KA, Krebs-Smith SM, Ballard-Barbash R, Cleveland LE. Food intakes of US children and adolescents compared with recommendations. Pediatrics 1997;100(3 Pt 1):323-329.

Murata M. Secular trends in growth and changes in eating patterns of Japanese children. Am J Clin Nutr 2000;72(5 Suppl):1379S-1383S.

Must A, Jacques PF, Dallal GE, Bajema CJ, Dietz WH. Long-term morbidity and mortality of overweight adolescents. A follow-up of the Harvard Growth Study of 1922 to 1935. N Engl J Med 1992;327(19):1350-1355.

Neuhouser ML, Kristal AR, Patterson RE. Use of food nutrition labels is associated with lower fat intake. J Am Diet Assoc 1999; 99(1):45-53.

Neumark-Sztainer D, Story M, Perry C, Casey MA. Factors influencing food choices of adolescents: findings from focus-group discussions with adolescents. J Am Diet Assoc 1999;99(8):929-937.

Nielsen SJ, Siega-Riz AM, Popkin BM. Trends in energy intake in U.S. between 1977 and 1996: Similar shifts seen across age groups. Obes Res 2002; 10(5):370-378.

Ogden CL, Flegal KM, Carroll MD, Johnson CL. Prevalence and trends in overweight among US children and adolescents, 1999-2000. JAMA 2002;288(14):1728-1732.

Painter JE, Wansink B, Hieggelke JB. How visibility and convenience influence candy consumption. Appetite 2002;38(3):237-238.

Pendergrast M. For God, Country and Coca-Cola: The Definitive History of the Great American Soft Drink and the Company that Makes It. New York, NY: Basic Books, 2000.

Pierce JW, Wardle J. Self-esteem, parental appraisal and body size in children. J Child Psychol Psychiatry 1993;34(7):1125-1136.

Pierce JW, Wardle J. Cause and effect beliefs and self-esteem of overweight children. J Child Psychol Psychiatry 1997; 38(6):645-650.

Pine DS, Goldstein RB, Wolk S, Weissman MM. The association between childhood depression and adulthood body mass index. Pediatrics 2001;107(5):1049-1056.

Pinhas-Hamiel O, Dolan LM, Daniels SR, Standiford D, Khoury PR, Zeitler P. Increased incidence of non-insulin-dependent diabetes mellitus among adolescents. J Pediatr 1996;128 (5 Pt 1):608-615.

Poirier P, Despres JP. Obesity and cardiovascular disease. Med Sci (Paris) 2003;19(10):943-949.

Pollak CP, Bright D. Caffeine consumption and weekly sleep patterns in US seventh-, eighth-, and ninth-graders. Pediatrics 2003;111(1):42-46.

Popkin BM, Nielsen SJ. The sweetening of the world's diet. Obes Res 2003;11(11):1325-1332.

Proctor MH, Moore LL, Gao D, Cupples LA, Bradlee ML, Hood MY et al. Television viewing and change in body fat from preschool to early adolescence: The Framingham Children's Study. Int J Obes Relat Metab Disord 2003; 7(7):827-833.

Putnam J, Gerrior S. Trends in the US Food Supply, 1970–97. USDA Chapter 7, Report: AIB-750.

Redline S, Tishler PV, Schluchter M, Aylor J, Clark K, Graham G. Risk factors for sleep-disordered breathing in children. Associations with obesity, race, and respiratory problems. Am J Respir Crit Care Med 1999;159(5 Pt 1):1527-1532.

Rhodes SK, Shimoda KC, Waid LR, O'Neil PM, Oexmann MJ, Collop NA et al. Neurocognitive deficits in morbidly obese children with obstructive sleep apnea. J Pediatr 1995;127(5):741-744.

Robinson TN. Television viewing and childhood obesity. Pediatr Clin North Am 2001;48(4):1017-1025.

Rozin P, Kabnick K, Pete E, Fischler C, Shields C. The ecology of eating: Smaller portion sizes in France than in the United States help explain the French paradox. Psychol Sci 2003;14(5):450-454.

Rudolf MC, Greenwood DC, Cole TJ, Levine R, Sahota P, Walker J et al. Rising obesity and expanding waistlines in schoolchildren: A cohort study. Arch Dis Child 2004;89:235-237.

Saelens BE, Sallis JF, Black JB, Chen D. Neighborhood-based differences in physical activity: an environment scale evaluation. Am J Public Health 2003;93(9):1552-1558.

Salmeron J, Manson JE, Stampfer MJ, Colditz GA, Wing AL, Willett WC. Dietary fiber, glycemic load, and risk of non-insulin-dependent diabetes mellitus in women. JAMA 1997;277(6):472-477.

Schwartz MB, Chambliss HO, Brownell KD, Blair SN, Billington C. Weight bias among health professionals specializing in obesity. Obes Res 2003; 11(9):1033-1039.

Schwartz MB, Puhl R. Childhood obesity: A societal problem to solve. Obes Rev 2003;4(1):57-71.

Segal NL, Allison DB. Twins and virtual twins: Bases of relative body weight revisited. Int J Obes Relat Metab Disord 2002;26(4):437-441.

Sheslow D, Hassink S, Wallace W, DeLancey E. The relationship between self-esteem and depression in obese children. Ann N Y Acad Sci 1993;699:289-291.

Sinha R, Fisch G, Teague B, Tamborlane WV, Banyas B, Allen K et al. Prevalence of impaired glucose tolerance among children and adolescents with marked obesity. N Engl J Med 2002;346(11):802-810.

St John AT, Ogden J. What do mothers feed their children and why? Health Educ Res 1999;14(6):717-727.

Steinberger J, Moran A, Hong CP, Jacobs DR, Jr., Sinaiko AR. Adiposity in childhood predicts obesity and insulin resistance in young adulthood. J Pediatr 2001;138(4):469-473.

Stradmeijer M, Bosch J, Koops W, Seidell J. Family functioning and psychosocial adjustment in overweight youngsters. Int J Eat Disord 2000;27(1):110-114.

Strauss RS. Childhood obesity and self-esteem. Pediatrics 2000;105(1):e15.

Strauss RS, Barlow SE, Dietz WH. Prevalence of abnormal serum aminotransferase values in overweight and obese adolescents. J Pediatr 2000;136(6):727-733.

Strauss RS, Pollack HA. Social marginalization of overweight children. Arch Pediatr Adolesc Med 2003;157(8):746-752.

Sturm R. The effects of obesity, smoking, and drinking on medical problems and costs. Obesity outranks both smoking and drinking in its deleterious effects on health and health costs. Health Aff (Millwood) 2002;21(2):245-253.

Subar AF, Krebs-Smith SM, Cook A, Kahle LL. Dietary sources of nutrients among US children, 1989-1991. Pediatrics 1998;102(4 Pt 1):913-923.

Taras HL, Gage M. Advertised foods on children's television. Arch Pediatr Adolesc Med 1995;149(6):649-652.

Taras HL, Sallis JF, Patterson TL, Nader PR, Nelson JA. Television's influence on children's diet and physical activity. J Dev Behav Pediatr 1989;10(4):176-180.

Taylor RW, Jones IE, Williams SM, Goulding A. Evaluation of waist circumference, waist-to-hip ratio, and the conicity index as screening tools for high trunk fat mass, as measured by dual-energy X-ray absorptiometry, in children aged 3-19 y. Am J Clin Nutr 2000;72(2):490-495.

Thompson SH, Corwin SJ, Sargent RG. Ideal body size beliefs and weight concerns of fourth-grade children. Int J Eat Disord 1997;21(3):279-284.

Tippet KS, Cleveland LE. How Current diets stack up: Comparison with dietary guidelines. USDA Chapter 3, Report: AIB-750.

Toeller M, Buyken AE, Heitkamp G, Cathelineau G, Ferriss B, Michel G. Nutrient intakes as predictors of body weight in European people with type 1 diabetes. Int J Obes Relat Metab Disord 2001;25(12):1815-1822.

Tremblay MS, Katzmarzyk PT, Willms JD. Temporal trends in overweight and obesity in Canada, 1981-1996. Int J Obes Relat Metab Disord 2002;26(4):538-543.

Tremblay MS, Willms JD. Secular trends in the body mass index of Canadian children. CMAJ 2000;163(11):1429-1433.

Tsukada H, Miura K, Kido T, Saeki K, Kawashima H, Ikawa A et al. [Relationship of childhood obesity to adult obesity: a 20-year longitudinal study from birth in Ishikawa Prefecture, Japan]. Nippon Koshu Eisei Zasshi 2003;50(12):1125-1134.

Wallace WJ, Sheslow D, Hassink S. Obesity in children: A risk for depression. Ann N Y Acad Sci 1993;699:301-303.

Wang G, Dietz WH. Economic burden of obesity in youths aged 6 to 17 years: 1979-1999. Pediatrics 2002;109(5):E81.

Wang Y, Monteiro C, Popkin BM. Trends of obesity and underweight in older children and adolescents in the United States, Brazil, China, and Russia. Am J Clin Nutr 2002;75(6):971-977.

Wansink B. At the movies: How external cues and perceived taste impact consumption volume. Food Quality and Preference 2001;12(1):69-74.

Wardle J, Guthrie C, Sanderson S, Birch L, Plomin R. Food and activity preferences in children of lean and obese parents. Int J Obes Relat Metab Disord 2001;25(7):971-977.

Wardle J, Volz C, Golding C. Social variation in attitudes to obesity in children. Int J Obes Relat Metab Disord 1995;19(8):562-569.

Whitaker RC, Wright JA, Pepe MS, Seidel KD, Dietz WH. Predicting obesity in young adulthood from childhood and parental obesity. N Engl J Med 1997;337(13):869-873.

Index

More Great Books from Robert Rose

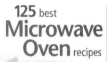

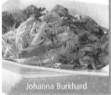

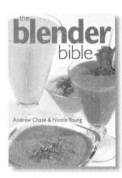

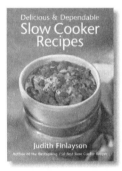

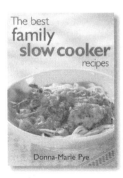

Appliance Cooking

- 125 Best Microwave Oven Recipes
  by Johanna Burkhard
- The Blender Bible
  by Andrew Chase and Nicole Young
- The Mixer Bible
  by Meredith Deeds and Carla Snyder
- The 150 Best Slow Cooker Recipes
  by Judith Finlayson
- Delicious & Dependable Slow Cooker Recipes
  by Judith Finlayson
- 125 Best Vegetarian Slow Cooker Recipes
  by Judith Finlayson
- 125 Best Rotisserie Oven Recipes
  by Judith Finlayson
- 125 Best Food Processor Recipes
  by George Geary
- The Best Family Slow Cooker Recipes
  by Donna-Marie Pye
- The Best Convection Oven Cookbook
  by Linda Stephen
- 125 Best Toaster Oven Recipes
  by Linda Stephen
- 250 Best American Bread Machine Baking Recipes
  by Donna Washburn and Heather Butt
- 250 Best Canadian Bread Machine Baking Recipes
  by Donna Washburn and Heather Butt

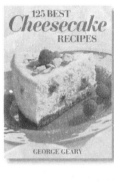

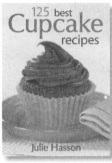

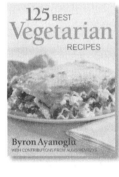

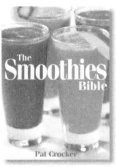

Baking

- 250 Best Cakes & Pies
  by Esther Brody
- 500 Best Cookies, Bars & Squares
  by Esther Brody
- 500 Best Muffin Recipes
  by Esther Brody
- 125 Best Cheesecake Recipes
  by George Geary
- 125 Best Chocolate Recipes
  by Julie Hasson
- 125 Best Chocolate Chip Recipes
  by Julie Hasson
- 125 Best Cupcake Recipes
  by Julie Hasson
- Complete Cake Mix Magic
  by Jill Snider

Healthy Cooking

- 125 Best Vegetarian Recipes
  by Byron Ayanoglu with contributions from Algis Kemezys
- America's Best Cookbook for Kids with Diabetes
  by Colleen Bartley
- Canada's Best Cookbook for Kids with Diabetes
  by Colleen Bartley
- The Juicing Bible
  by Pat Crocker and Susan Eagles
- The Smoothies Bible
  by Pat Crocker

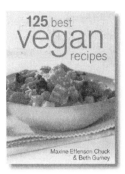

- 125 Best Vegan Recipes
  by Maxine Effenson Chuck and Beth Gurney
- 500 Best Healthy Recipes
  Edited by Lynn Roblin, RD
- 125 Best Gluten-Free Recipes
  by Donna Washburn and Heather Butt
- The Best Gluten-Free Family Cookbook
  by Donna Washburn and Heather Butt

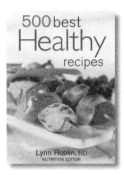

- America's Everyday Diabetes Cookbook
  Edited by Katherine E. Younker, MBA, RD
- Canada's Everyday Diabetes Choice Recipes
  Edited by Katherine E. Younker, MBA, RD
- Canada's Complete Diabetes Cookbook
  Edited by Katherine E. Younker, MBA, RD
- The Best Diabetes Cookbook (U.S.)
  Edited by Katherine E. Younker, MBA, RD
- The Best Low-Carb Cookbook
  from Robert Rose

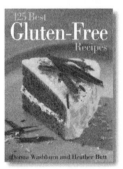

Recent Bestsellers

- 125 Best Soup Recipes
  by Marylin Crowley and Joan Mackie
- The Convenience Cook
  by Judith Finlayson
- 125 Best Ice Cream Recipes
  by Marilyn Linton and Tanya Linton

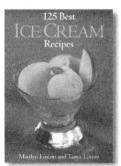

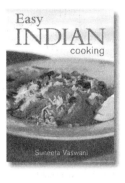

- Easy Indian Cooking
  by Suneeta Vaswani
- Simply Thai Cooking
  by Wandee Young and Byron Ayanoglu

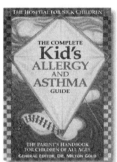

Health

- The Complete Natural Medicine Guide to the 50 Most Common Medicinal Herbs
  by Dr. Heather Boon, B.Sc.Phm., Ph.D., and Michael Smith, B.Pharm, M.R.Pharm.S., ND
- The Complete Kid's Allergy and Asthma Guide
  Edited by Dr. Milton Gold
- The Complete Natural Medicine Guide to Breast Cancer
  by Sat Dharam Kaur, ND

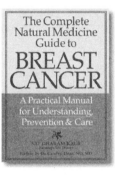

- The Complete Doctor's Stress Solution
  by Penny Kendall-Reed, MSc, ND, and Dr. Stephen Reed, MD, FRCSC
- The Complete Doctor's Healthy Back Bible
  by Dr. Stephen Reed, MD, and Penny Kendall-Reed, MSc, ND, with Dr. Michael Ford, MD, FRCSC, and Dr. Charles Gregory, MD, ChB, FRCP(C)

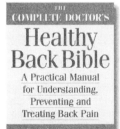

- Everyday Risks in Pregnancy & Breastfeeding
  by Dr. Gideon Koren, MD, FRCP(C), ND
- Help for Eating Disorders
  by Dr. Debra Katzman, MD, FRCP(C), and Dr. Leora Pinhas, MD

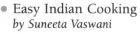

Also Available
from Robert Rose

THE COMPLETE GUIDE TO
Everyday Risks
in
Pregnancy
&
Breastfeeding

❋ ❋ ❋ ❋ ❋

Answers To Your Questions
About Morning Sickness,
Medications, Herbs, Diseases,
Chemical Exposures & More

Dr. Gideon Koren, MD, FRCP(C)

FROM THE **MOTHERISK** PROGRAM AT
THE HOSPITAL FOR SICK CHILDREN

ISBN: 0-7788-0084-9 / $24.95 Canada / $17.95 U.S.

For more great books, see previous pages

Robert
ROSE